T0326340

A Practical Guide to Portable Pupillometry

"Merlin Larson is the world's authority on pupils and anesthesia and has spent his life studying this fascinating and underappreciated window into the brain. In this monograph, Professor Larson presents an engaging non-technical history of the pupil and clearly explains how pupillary measurements have improved our understanding of anesthesia. It is well worth reading!"

Daniel I. Sessler, MD, Professor and
Michael Cudahy Chair, Outcomes Research Consortium,
Cleveland Clinic

"Merlin Larson absolutely nails this practical guide to portable pupillometry, setting the tone and capturing the reader with the fascinating history of thoughts on the pupil as a window to the soul, the heart, and the brain. Professor Larson brings his decades-long journey, in the fashion of his former colleague, John Severinghaus, to describe how he and others have created this important tool and its many practical applications in perioperative and critical care medicine. The large majority of this book provides fundamental concepts of anatomy, circuitry, physiology, and pharmacology, which are presented in an easy-to-understand manner without talking down to the reader. The book succeeds in being extremely up to date while taking pains to include how this tool is likely to evolve in the near future. As a researcher who utilizes desktop pupillometry on a regular basis, I learned much from this book and wish it had been available when I first started study of this fascinating structure."

James C. Eisenach, M.D., F.M. James, III Professor
of Anesthesiology,
Wake Forest University School of Medicine,
Winston-Salem, North Carolina

"Portable pupillometry is increasingly being used as a diagnostic tool in clinical practice and holds tremendous promise to further expand our abilities to monitor central nervous function. However, until now, this tool was missing a guidebook that would inform the interested practitioner about the underlying science. Few users of infrared pupillometry are aware about its diagnostic possibilities and limitations, or know about its many established – and potential future – clinical applications. *A Practical Guide to Portable Pupillometry* closes this gap, serving both as an introduction to the field and as a reference for the experienced clinician or researcher using pupillometry."

Merlin Larson established himself during his long scientific career as the leading expert in the field of portable pupillometry. His pioneering work laid the foundations of pupillometry use in anesthesia, pain management, and resuscitation. *A Practical Guide to Portable Pupillometry* gives the reader access to Dr. Larson's vast knowledge in an exciting, expanding field of clinical care and scientific exploration."

Matthias Behrends, MD, Health Science Clinical Professor,
and Medical Director of Inpatient Pain Services,
Department of Anesthesia and Perioperative Care,
University of California, San Francisco (UCSF)

A Practical Guide to Portable Pupillometry

Merlin D. Larson
University of California, San Francisco

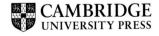
CAMBRIDGE
UNIVERSITY PRESS

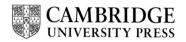

Shaftesbury Road, Cambridge CB2 8EA, United Kingdom

One Liberty Plaza, 20th Floor, New York, NY 10006, USA

477 Williamstown Road, Port Melbourne, VIC 3207, Australia

314–321, 3rd Floor, Plot 3, Splendor Forum, Jasola District Centre, New Delhi – 110025, India

103 Penang Road, #05–06/07, Visioncrest Commercial, Singapore 238467

Cambridge University Press is part of Cambridge University Press & Assessment, a department of the University of Cambridge.

We share the University's mission to contribute to society through the pursuit of education, learning and research at the highest international levels of excellence.

www.cambridge.org
Information on this title: www.cambridge.org/9781009436298

DOI: 10.1017/9781009436274

First published 2025

A catalogue record for this publication is available from the British Library.

A Cataloging-in-Publication data record for this book is available from the Library of Congress.

ISBN 978-1-009-43629-8 Paperback

....

About the Author

The author studied at the National Institutes of Health and Stanford University. Following his anesthesia training, he was Chairman of the Department of Anesthesia at French Hospital, San Francisco and Clinical Instructor at the University of California, San Francisco. In 1989, he joined the full-time faculty at the University of California, San Francisco and is now Professor Emeritus of Anesthesiology and Peri-Operative Medicine. He served as Chief of the Acute Pain Service at Mount Zion Hospital in San Francisco from 2013 to 2019. He has studied pupillary behavior during anesthesia for over 40 years and has published extensively on the topic. In 2001, he hosted the International Pupil Colloquium at Asilomar, California.

Contents

Preface

As a medical student, I wanted to study neurotransmission in the brain. At the time, in 1965, this was an emerging new science based on how neurons communicated with each other. It was an exciting time because John Eccles had recently detected acetylcholine-mediated transmission in the spinal cord, and various amino acids were also candidates as central neurotransmitters (1, 2).

The Chair of the Pharmacology Department at the University of Kansas, Edward J. Walaszek, was attracted by my interest because of his research on the cataleptic bulbocapnine. He accepted me into a summer project to study how alterations in brain catecholamine levels changed the cataleptic response to bulbocapnine. My research went through two summers and the data was later published in manuscripts by Drs. Walaszek and John Chapman (3). The tentative conclusion that bulbocapnine interfered with dopamine neurotransmission has more recently been studied by other investigators (4).

These questions about neurotransmission in the central nervous system remained on my mind during my internship year at the Hospital of the University of Pennsylvania. My mentors that year promoted my continued involvement in this topic and gave me recommendations to continue my studies at the National Institutes of Health under the direct supervision of Drs. G. C. Salmoiraghi, Forrest Weight, and Floyd Bloom. Dr. Salmoiraghi had perfected a method of recording electrical potentials inside central neurons while giving drugs through a glass pipette on the outside of the same neuron (5).

My initial mentor in that lab was Forrest Weight, who was recording electrical potentials inside the large motoneurons of the cat spinal cord. Because anesthetics interfere with drug effects in the brain, his studies were performed without anesthesia. Cats were anesthetized with ether and a mid-collicular *cerveau isole* was electrolytically performed on the anesthetized animal. When the ether was discontinued, these animals would tolerate the surgical procedure of exposing the spinal cord without distress. Our reassuring sign was an animal with tightly constricted pupils who was not responsive to surgical stimulation. Failing that, we would abandon the case or attempt another mid-collicular *cerveau isole* preparation. The papers by F. Bremer from the 1930s (6) pointed to an area in the reticular formation below the nucleus of the third cranial nerve as the target of our electrolytic lesions that resulted in favorable conditions for our experiments without anesthetic agents.

In 1966, Dr. Weight left the laboratory for a two-year sabbatical in Sweden. I continued the same feline study by myself, but with a question regarding the neurotransmitters that excite and inhibit the motoneuron. The motoneuron was inhibited by a feedback mechanism. Strychnine blocked the inhibition, but how it did so was not known. These experiments showed that strychnine blocked the inhibitions elicited by glycine, but not those elicited by GABA (7) (Figure 0.1), lending support to the theory that the convulsant action of strychnine was brought about by antagonizing glycine inhibition. Because glycine is located predominantly in the spinal cord, the convulsions are primarily in the limbs, and the subjects are often awake during the convulsion. The studies at NIH introduced me to the phenomena of inhibitory mechanisms in the brain, a topic that has continued to interest me throughout my career.

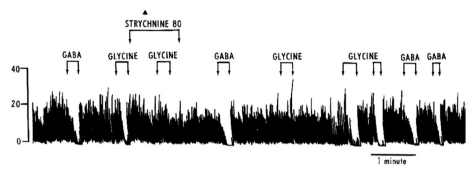

Figure 0.1 Iontophoretic application of GABA and glycine onto a motoneuron in the cat spinal cord. Note that strychnine blocked the inhibition of glycine, but not the inhibition of GABA (7). The following pages will explain how inhibitory transmission in the mesencephalon plays a major role in the control of pupil size and reactivity. Permission from Elsevier to reproduce image, License Number: 5593111219239.

My final project at NIH was to measure the effect of a barbiturate, hexobarbital, on the recurrent inhibitory process that is produced by activation of the Renshaw cells. My colleague Mitchell Major and I observed an intensification of this inhibition and published it in a short report in *Brain Research* in 1969. This observation led us to speculate that anesthetics might act partially by intensifying inhibition in the CNS (8).

The management of performing surgical procedures on cats without any anesthetic agents was challenging. The portions of the brain stem that required ablation for the *cerveau isole* preparation led me into thinking about the neurophysiology of anesthesia. John Bunker was Chair of the anesthesia department at Stanford and had similar interests. He recruited me into the anesthesia residency at Stanford University Hospital in 1968. We both felt that pursuing the questions surrounding inhibitory processes in the brain had implications for the mechanisms of anesthesia.

As I progressed through residency, the thought of the miotic pupil of the *cerveau isole* preparation resurfaced. But measuring the pupil during anesthesia presented a problem. Seventy-five years ago, there were many comments about the size of the pupil and its reactivity to light in books relating to anesthesia and critical care (9). Noticeably lacking were any actual numbers that documented the changes that were said to occur. For example, the original papers of Guedel (9), Gillespie, Poe (10), Clement, and others demonstrated charts that showed black circles that were supposed to represent the changes that were brought about by anesthetics, pain, and analgesics. Cullen and others positioned a mm rule next to the orbit, and this method provided a crude measure of pupil size, but did not measure the dynamic reflexes of constriction and dilation (11). The classic book by Plum and Posner on coma had extensive discussions on the pupil, but they did not include quantitative measurements (12).

On the other hand, Irene Loewenfeld had precisely measured pupillary reactivity relating to drugs and to critical events in animals and humans. These precise measurements were taken with a new technology using infrared light, thus avoiding the confounding effects of visible light on the pupil. The Loewenfeld records documented that the mechanism of pupillary reflex dilation was brought about through different mechanisms in the awake compared to the anesthetized animal (13). A discussion of reflex dilation will be presented in later chapters. The only academic work on the effect of anesthetics and opioids on the pupil in humans at that time had been performed by measuring the pupil with calipers or a mm rule (11, 14).

None of these prior discussions of pupillary reactivity would fit with what was observed during a typical anesthetic that was being used during the early 1970s. The newer halogenated agents like halothane did not produce the same changes in the pupil as had been described for ether. It seemed like a simple project to measure the pupil during the typical anesthetic of meperidine, thiopental, halothane, nitrous oxide, curare, neostigmine, and atropine. However, a pupillometer was not a device that was available in anesthesia departments. Frederic Hewitt (1857–1916) had made a crude pupil gauge and Cullen and others had used a mm rule positioned next to the eye (11). I was motivated to make a simple dot comparison pupillometer with an attached magnifying glass to evaluate the size and light reaction during induction of anesthesia with thiopental. Initial studies with this device were published in *Anesthesiology Review* (15) and attracted the attention of three retired executives of the DuPont Company who were interested in the detection of opioid abuse with pupillometry. They suggested that I help them construct a portable infrared pupillometer that would be an objective measure of pupillary size and pupillary reactions. Their company was named Fairville Medical Optics after the location near the DuPont mansion in Fairville, PA. The Fairville pupillometers went through several iterations and eventually were developed into an instrument that was able to measure and record without requiring a connecting laptop computer. These instruments will be discussed in more detail in Chapter 6.

In 1989, Peter Brock, the director of Fairville Medical Optics, visited me in San Francisco and we showed the Fairville pupillometer to Larry Stark at the University of California, Berkeley. Dr Stark was the expert in measuring the pupil with infrared light (16), but he had not considered the idea of developing a portable instrument. A new company later built on the idea of a portable instrument and invented the Neuroptics pupillometers, which became available in 1995.

These developments led to the idea of using accurate pupillary measurements in the areas of anesthesia and critical care. Consequently, I attended several sessions of the "Pupil Colloquium" where the experts on the pupil from various disciplines meet to discuss the clinical applications of pupillary measurements. At these meetings, I became acquainted with Irene Loewenfeld, Stan Thompson, Elemer Szabadi, Stuart Steinhauer, Barbara Wilhelm, Helmut Wilhelm, Paul Gamlin, Dion Bremner, Steven Smith, and Randy Kardon. In learning about the effect of anesthetics on the pupil, I became aware of how little was known about the pupil by the average physician.

In 1989, the hospital where I practiced closed and I was able to secure a position as an attending physician in the Anesthesiology Department at the University of California, San Francisco. This change in employment initiated a series of studies on the pupil that have continued to this day. I conducted several studies between the years 1990 and 2000 in collaboration with Daniel Sessler, who was studying the effect of anesthetics on thermoregulation (17). It was easy to devise a pupillary project to integrate into these studies. The questions at that time were related to the effects of hypnotics and analgesics on three separate parameters: pupil diameter (PD), pupillary light reflex (PLR), and pupillary reflex dilation (PRD). With the use of the Fairville pupillometer, we documented that the dilation of the pupil that followed a nociceptive stimulus was more robust than the hemodynamic measures that responded to the same stimulus (18).

The neurophysiology of the pupil is complex. It is poorly understood by many physicians. It became apparent that writing articles about pupillary physiology would have little impact because of this lack of understanding. To propose ideas to the wider medical community it seemed necessary first to put together a monograph outlining the rationale for measuring the pupil. This book attempts to achieve that goal, but it is not intended to be the final word on any topic. To facilitate the ease of reading the text and economize on space, the author has omitted tables and statistical treatments. Tables and statistical data can be found by reading the referenced manuscripts. The book begins with a historical summary about the pupil and from there slowly builds a case for pupillary measurements to be used as a tool to impact clinical care. There will be mistakes in this narrative and the author would be delighted to receive comments on any aspect of the book (merlin.larson@ucsf.edu).

The author is not affiliated with or funded by commercial entities. The ideas are my own and will provoke controversy. But valid disagreements will ultimately lead to a more complete understanding of this new technology. With time, these discussions will clearly define the circumstances where pupillometry can be a useful addition to medical science.

Acknowledgements

The author is indebted to the following individuals with whom discussions about the pupil have contributed to the contents of this book: Thierry Bagnol, Matthias Behrends, Kumar Belani, Peter Berry, Michael Bokoch, Peter Brock, Elliot Carter, Peter Cheng, David Crankshaw, Malcolm Daniel, E. I. Eger, 2nd, Helge Eilers, James Eisenach, Antoine Elyn, Rachel Eshima-McKay, Pedro Gambus, Andrew Gray, Dhanesh Gupta, Claude Hemphill II, Ping Hill, Siddhartha Joshi, Randy Kardon, Evan Kharasch, Michael Kohn, Daniel Kondziella, Michael Koss, Andrea Kurz, Kate Leslie, Isabel Muhiudeen, Andrew Neice, Claus Niemann, Remi Pouchier, Claudio Privitera, Anthony Scott, Daniel Sessler, Kamran Siminou, Vineeta Singh, Wade Smith, Larry Stark, Stuart Steinhauer, Elemer Szabadi, Pekka Talke, Stanley Thompson, Sergio Vide, Barbara Wilhelm, and Helmut Wilhelm. Finally, I am grateful to Irene Loewenfeld with whom I had several conversations about the pupil. Irene Loewenfeld passed away in 2009.

Glossary

Accommodation: Adjustment of shape of the lens to optimize vision.

ACLS: Advanced cardiac life support.

Adrenalin: Epinephrine.

Afferent: A nerve impulse carrying a signal toward another nerve.

Algiscan: A pupillometer made by ID Med located in Marseille, France, that can stimulate selected dermatomes.

Algorithm: An ordered set of computerized instructions.

Ambient light: Normal indoor lighting, from 250 to 450 lux.

Amine: An organic compound that is a derivative of ammonia.

ANI: Analgesia Nociception Index. A measure of nociception during general anesthesia.

Anisocoria: Difference in size between the right and left pupils.

AU: Pupillary unrest in ambient light (PUAL) is measured in arbitrary units (AUs). This value reflects both the frequency and amplitude of the fluctuations of the pupil when exposed to light.

Bilateral: On both sides of the body.

Blocked dermatomes: Dermatomes that lack sensation because of a regional block.

BMI: Body mass index, considered to be a rough measure of body fat.

Brain stem: Portion of the central nervous system between the thalamus and the spinal cord.

Camera obscura: A dark space containing a small hole through which an image can be projected on a screen.

Cataract: An opacity in the lens of the eye.

Catecholamine: An organic compound containing a catechol group. Some of the catecholamine neurotransmitters in the brain are epinephrine, norepinephrine, and dopamine.

Caudal: A neuraxial block by injection of local anesthetics into the sacral hiatus.

Cephalad: Toward the head.

Cerveau isole: An operation that transects the midbrain below the oculomotor nucleus.

CNS: Central nervous system.

Coma: A state of unresponsiveness with eyes closed and unresponsive to vigorous stimulation.

Consensual reflex: The constriction of the pupil when light is directed into the opposite pupil.

Contralateral: On the opposite side.

CPR: Cardiopulmonary resuscitation.

CSF: Cerebral spinal fluid.

CVP: Central venous pressure.

Delirium: A temporary disorder of mental faculties.

Denervation: Loss of nerve supply to an area of the body.

Dermatome: The sensory area innervated by one spinal segment.

Desynchronized sleep: Sleep during which EEG resembles the awake condition.

Diplopia: Double vision.

Dot comparison pupillometer: A pupillometer consisting of different sizes of circular black dots.

Drug tolerance: A decrease in drug effect after prolonged use.

ECMO: Extracorporeal membrane oxygenation. A method to support the circulation and gas exchange in persons whose heart and lungs are unable to support life.

EEG: Electroencephalogram.

Efferent: A nerve impulse carrying a message away from another nerve.

EKG: Electrocardiogram.

Electromechanical dissociation: Lack of cardiac function with continuation of cardiac electrical activity.

Endoscopy: Insertion of a thin tube into the body to visualize an internal organ.

Epidural: A regional block produced by injection of agents into the epidural space.

Etiology: Pertaining to the cause of an event.

EW: Edinger Westphal nucleus. A region in the upper midbrain that contains the neurons that initiate the pupillary light reflex.

EWcp: The portion of the Edinger Westphal nucleus that projects centrally and is not involved in generating the pupillary light reflex.

EWpg: Preganglionic Edinger Westphal neurons that provide the nicotinic cholinergic input to the ciliary ganglion. These neurons generate the pupillary light reflex.

Extramission: The theory that vision is brought about by eye beams emitted from the eye.

Extubation: Removal of a tracheal tube.

FFT: Fast Fourier Transform. A mathematical operation that separates a fluctuating signal into frequency and amplitude components.

Fluctuation: An irregular chaotic change in the size of the pupil.

fMRI: Functional magnetic resonance imaging. An imaging method that demonstrates changes in brain metabolism.

Four Score: A 16-point scale that indicates the severity of neurological impairment.

GABA: Gamma aminobutyric acid. An inhibitory transmitter in the brain.

General anesthesia: An anesthetic that includes loss of consciousness.

Glasgow coma scale (GCS): A 15-point scale that indicates the severity of functional neurological impairment.

ICP: Intracranial pressure.

ICU: Intensive Care Unit.

Illumination: The intensity of light falling on a given surface. The Neuroptics PLR-3000 device provides the energy delivered to the LEDs in microwatts. Approximate illuminations are as follows: 10 microwatts: 80 lux, 50 microwatts: 410 lux, 121 microwatts: 1,000 lux, 180 microwatts, 1,500 lux. The NPi-300 and the Neurolight illuminate at approximately 1,000 lux.

Infrared: A type of electromagnetic radiation with a wavelength that is longer than visible light.

Inhibition: A type of neurotransmission in the brain that inhibits the activity of other neurons.

Intracranial: Within the cranium.

Intraoperative: Occurring during an operation.

Intromission: The theory that vision is brought about by light rays entering the pupil.

ipRGCs: Intrinsic photosensitive retinal ganglion cells. Retinal ganglion cells that respond to light in the absence of rod and cone photoreceptors.

LC: Locus coeruleus. A brain stem nucleus in the pons containing norepinephrine.

Limbus: The junction between the cornea and the sclera of the eye.

LO: Light off. An abrupt change from brightness to darkness.

LSD: Lysergic acid diethylamide. A synthetic potent psychedelic drug.

MAC: Minimum anesthetic concentration, a measure of anesthetic potency.

Medulla: The lowest portion of the brain, which connects it to the spinal cord.

Midbrain: The uppermost portion of the brain stem.

Miosis: A small constricted pupil, below 3 mm in diameter in dim light.

Motoneuron: Large neurons in the spinal cord that innervate muscles to initiate movement.

MRI: Magnetic resonance imaging. A noninvasive process that produces detailed images of the body.

Near vision: Viewing objects close to the face.

Neuraxial block: A regional block by injecting local anesthetics into the neuraxis.

Neurolight: A pupillometer made by ID Med located in Marseille, France that is designed to measure the light reflex and PUAL.

Neuromuscular blocking agent: A drug like curare that paralyzes skeletal muscles.

Neuroptics: A company located in Laguna Hills, CA that makes pupillometers.

Neurotransmission: The process of transferring messages in the brain.

Neurotransmitter: A chemical that is released by a nerve to activate or inhibit another nerve or muscle.

NMDA antagonist: A drug like ketamine that blocks the N-methyl-D-aspartate receptor.

Nociception: The physiological response to activation of nociceptors.

Nociceptor: A specialized receptor that responds to intense stimuli that are potentially harmful.

NOL: Nociception Level. A monitor designed to objectively quantify pain and nociception.

NPi: Neurological Pupil index. An algorithm proposed by Neuroptics, Inc. to evaluate the quality of the pupillary light reflex.

NSAIDs: Nonsteroidal anti-inflammatory drugs. A non-opioid alternative for treatment of pain.

Ophthalmoscope: An instrument that permits visualization through the pupil into the interior of the eye.

Opioid: A natural or synthetic drug derived from opium.

Optic nerve: The second cranial nerve that transmits the visual sensation to the brain

PACU: Post-Anesthesia Care Unit

Pain: An unpleasant sensory and emotional response to real or imagined tissue injury.

Palpebral fissure: The open space between the upper and lower eyelids.

Parameter: A measurement that can be given a specific value.

Parasympathetic: That portion of the autonomic nervous system that arises from cranial and sacral nerves.

PCA: Patient controlled analgesia. The patient controls a pump that delivers analgesics.

PD: Pupil diameter.

PET scan: Positron emission tomography. An imaging technique that uses radioactive tracers to detect disease at an early stage of development.

Photopigment: A pigment in the retina whose chemical state depends on the degree of illumination.

Photoreceptor: Neurons in the retina that convert light into electrical neuronal signals.

PIPR: Post Illumination Pupillary Response. A sustained pupillary constriction following short wavelength light stimulation.

PLR: Pupillary light reflex.

Pons: That portion of the brain stem that lies between the medulla oblongata and the midbrain.

PPI: Pupillary Pain Index. A pupillometric technique designed to detect intraoperative analgesia.

PRD: Pupillary Reflex Dilation.

PUAL: Pupillary unrest in ambient light. The strength of the pupillary fluctuations in ambient light.

PUI: Pupillary Unrest Index. A long duration measurement of pupil size that is proposed to detect drowsiness.

Pupillometer: An electronic device that measures the pupil.

Pupillometry: The process of using pupillometers to measure the pupil and its reactions.

QPi: Quality of the pupillary light reflex. A number generated by the Neurolight pupillometers to gauge the quality of the pupillary light reflex.

Radial muscle: The radial muscle is the dilator muscle of the iris that is innervated by the sympathetic nervous system.

RAPD: Relative afferent pupillary defect. A relative defect in transmitting light excitation from the retina to the olivary pretectal nucleus as compared to the opposite side.

RASS: Richmond Agitation–Sedation Scale, a measure of sedation or agitation. Plus 4 is very combative and minus 5 is unarousable sedation.

Receptor: A specialized portion of a neuron that is activated by a neurotransmitter.

Regional block: Local anesthetic induced loss of sensation.

Reticular formation: A complex group of neurons in the brain stem that are crucial for maintaining a state of consciousness.

ROSC: Return of spontaneous circulation.

RR interval: The time elapsed between two successive R waves on the electrocardiogram.

Sensitivity: The ability of a test to correctly designate a person as positive for a condition such as disease state.

Smooth muscles: Involuntary muscles innervated by the autonomic nervous system in the hollow organs, the iris, and the walls of blood vessels.

Specificity: The ability of a test to give a negative result in a person who is actually negative for a condition.

SPI: Surgical Pleth Index. An objective measure of nociception that uses plethysmographic signals.

Strabismus: A disorder of the extraocular muscles so that both eyes cannot fixate on the same object.

Subcortical: That portion of the brain that is below the cortex.

Supraspinal: The central nervous system above the spinal cord.

Sympathetic nervous system: A portion of the autonomic nervous system that arises from the first thoracic segment to the second lumbar segment.

Synapse: A specialized junction between two neurons that can be activated by a neurotransmitter.

Synchronized sleep: Slow-wave sleep.

TBI: Traumatic brain injury.

Tetanic stimulus: A painful electrical stimulus applied to the skin, typically stimulating at 50 to 100 Hz.

THC: Tetrahydrocannabinol. The principle psychoactive ingredient in cannabis.

TIVA: Total intravenous anesthesia. General anesthesia that is produced only via the intravenous route.

Toxic dose: A dose of a drug that is either lethal or nearly lethal.

Tracheal intubation: Insertion of a breathing tube into the trachea.

UCSF: University of California, San Francisco.

Ultrasound: A technique that uses high-frequency sound waves to make images of structures within the body.

Unilateral: One-sided.

Ventilation: Spontaneous or mechanically assisted breathing.

Vertex distance: The distance from the front surface of the cornea to the lens of the optical device.

Volatile anesthetic: An inhaled anesthetic that is a vapor.

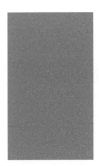

Introduction

The gods put in a face in which they inserted organs to minister in all things
to the providence of the soul. They first contrived the eyes, into which they
conveyed a light akin to the light of day, making it flow through the pupils.

(Plato, *Timaeus*)

The brain is the organ of perception and cognition and so it is understandable that it is
studied by thousands of scientists around the world. But the brain is encased in solid
bone, making it difficult to study. We can't see, probe, or touch it without major surgery,
so we often rely on indirect methods such as personal interviews or autonomic measures
such as heart rate or blood pressure. Other techniques to study the brain require
expensive specialized equipment such as electroencephalograms, fMRI, PET scans, or
magnetoencephalograms.

Fortunately, one tiny piece of the human brain is visible. The pupil is the opening in
the center of the colored iris of the eye. The movements of the pupil are controlled by
muscles that are embryologically related to the central nervous system. Consequently,
modern techniques use the pupil to uncover useful information about the brain that was
not possible with older methods.

Our understanding of the pupil has taken over 3,000 years to develop and is continuing. Several prominent scientists of the past have been intrigued by the pupil. Archimedes
(287–212 BCE) devised a method to measure pupil diameter. In the seventeenth century,
the famous astronomer Galileo Galilei (1564–1642) developed his own technique to
estimate the size of the pupil. Descartes, Plato, Aristotle, Galen, and Scheiner all weighed
in with their thoughts about the pupil. Leonardo da Vinci (1452–1519) was fascinated by
the pupil. In his monograph on optics, he states the following: "O wonderful,
O marvelous necessity, you (the pupil) constrain with your laws all the effects to
participate in their causes in the most economical manner!! These are miracles!" (19, 20).

The opportunity to study the pupil scientifically was not possible until the late
twentieth century. Strict attention and proper methods of measurement during this
portion of the physical examination can provide useful information to the careful
examiner. "Proper methods of measurement" does not necessarily mean a desktop
pupillometer that can average several small responses to a repeated stimulus. With
those expensive instruments, it is possible to detect minuscule pupillary size changes to
attentional states because the instruments can use averaging techniques to extract small,
evoked responses of the pupil out of chaotic pupillary movements.

For the physician who wants to examine the pupillary reactions, there is a middle
ground between the office-based pupillometer and the naked eye examination. Portable

hand-held infrared pupillometers are an outgrowth of the technology that revolutionized the study of the pupil in the 1970s. These instruments are now located in many emergency rooms, operating rooms, and intensive care units around the world. They provide data on the pupillary light reflex (PLR), pupillary reflex dilation (PRD), and pupillary unrest in ambient light (PUAL). Light reflex amplitude, constriction velocity, dilation velocity, and latency of the reflex are other parameters that can be retrieved from the portable instruments. Interpretation of these parameters is required to extract useful information that pertains to care of the patient.

The pupillary light reflex is an important segment of the physical examination. It therefore seems obvious that measurement of the reflex should provide accurate information. The problem with the traditional pen-light examination of the pupil is that over 50 percent of the world population have dark eyes. This means that to view the pupil, a high level of ambient light must be directed into or across the plane of the iris. Not only can adding this light confound the assessment of pupil size, because this ambient light constricts the pupil, but also, the important pupillary reflexes (light reflex and reflex dilation) are altered depending on the amount of light directed into the pupillary aperture. Infrared pupillometry can add value to these pupillary measures because the infrared light that illuminates the pupil does not alter pupil size or elicit a light reflex. There are several other issues that can confound the pen-light examination of pupil size and pupillary reflexes. The visual acuity of the examiner can be a factor. Also, the ambient light in the room, near fixation, extraneous alerting stimuli, and different examiners can all alter the assessment of the pupil. For these reasons, it is important to have a consistent method of pupillary examination, not only for the pen-light examination, but also when using the portable infrared instruments. Much of the valuable information that arises from measuring the pupil comes from trending the size and reactions over several hours or days. Clearly, if the measurements are done differently, then the trend becomes meaningless. The pupil can provide other information on the effect of drugs and neuropathology by recording the degree of pupillary unrest and pupillary reflex dilation.

The pupil has been and is continuing to be studied by several branches of medical and physical sciences. There are several hundred peer-reviewed manuscripts on the pupil published each year. As medical scientists become more and more specialized, their language and word usage take on specific meanings that are only completely understood by colleagues within the same specialty. Consequently, when an ophthalmologist interacts with a specialist in intensive care medicine and they discuss the pupil, certain sentences fail to convey their intended meaning. For example, a neurologist's use of the term "relative afferent defect" might go completely unnoticed by the pulmonologist who is directing the care of the patient, and this oversight might have important clinical ramifications. One method by which to correct this miscommunication is to examine the terms that have been used historically to describe pupillary behavior. Hopefully these specialized terms will then be more easily transferred across specialties so that more comprehensive discussions can take place.

Life and death, awareness, cognition, sensation, perception, anxiety, pain, and drug intoxication ... these are the issues that physicians contend with daily. The pupil and its reflexes can provide useful information on many of these topics. However, unless the practitioner admits that there is a problem with the evaluation of pupillary reflexes as it is often performed, then there will be little motivation to use a newer technology that can provide valuable data affecting the care of patients.

Before proceeding, certain facts about the portable infrared pupillary measurements should be made clear. First, it is not possible at the present time to measure the pupil continuously. Second, it is not possible to extract meaningful information through the closed eyelid. Ultrasound images of the pupil have been reported that can detect the presence or absence of the light reflex (21), but these methods have not yet been confirmed. In the future there might be methods that will be able to measure the pupil through the closed eyelid, but for now the cornea must be exposed. Third, midbrain and spinal cord clusters of neurons control the pupillary movements, so a functioning cerebral cortex is not necessary for pupillary reactions to be present. There are cortical influences on the pupillary light reflexes that will be discussed later, but the presence or absence of the reflex depends entirely on subcortical pathways. If the clinician understands how the pupil is controlled from the central nervous system, then at appropriate times these measurements can be taken, and useful information can be obtained. Finally, these instruments can measure the presence or absence of the consensual reflex, but giving a precise value to that reflex is not possible. It is possible to stimulate one eye with a pen light and measure the reflex in the opposite pupil with the portable instrument set at a zero-background light intensity. The stimulating light would vary between different measurements, so the light intensity would not always be the same. A modification of the Neuroptics pupillometer was described 20 years ago that would measure the consensual reflex with a portable pupillometer, but it is not commercially available at this time (22).

The normal human pupil ranges in diameter from 3 to 5 mm and over a daily 24-hour cycle may change from 2 to 8 mm. No other autonomic measure exhibits such a wide range of activity. The pupil fluctuates widely during periods of fatigue and in the interval just before sleep. It is miotic during slow-wave sleep and dilates during arousal and in darkness. Pupillary reactivity is maintained throughout the day and night. This is the normal behaving pupil.

During critical illness, there are factors that interrupt this normal behavior. These factors include the use of drugs that alter pupil size and reactivity, and the interruption of normal circadian rhythms. These changes in pupillary behavior are predictable and are well known to the average practitioner. Some pupillary changes, however, are outside the normal range of what is expected and thus represent erratic behavior. For example, 15 mg of intravenous morphine should produce a miotic pupil in the range of 2 to 3 mm as measured in darkness. If this does not occur, it would raise certain diagnostic questions regarding that patient (see Chapter 12). The pupil therefore provides information about the patient that might otherwise go undetected. Several other examples of how pupillary signs can assist the physician in the safe management of patients will be discussed in the following pages. Of primary importance is a thorough understanding of the light reflex and pupillary reflex dilation, the two basic pupillary reflexes.

This monograph traces the historical development of our present-day understanding of the pupil as it relates to the clinical practice of acute medicine. It is also a clinical guide to the diagnosis and interpretation of pupillary behavior in the hospital and office setting. It is not a book for the neuro-ophthalmologist who can study the pupil with specialized equipment in the office. Therefore, the author has purposely not emphasized several techniques used by the neuro-ophthalmologist such as the slit lamp and large office-based pupillometers. Also, the author will not discuss the detailed clinical use of many of the topical medications such as cocaine, methamphetamine, dapiprazole, brimonidine, and dopamine. Except for special clinical situations, these methods are omitted because other books provide a thorough treatment of this subject, and in the acute setting their use can result in anisocorias that further complicate evaluation of the patient.

New information about the pupil in the past 10 years has enabled the author to emphasize points that are not commonly known by many physicians. The book is intended to review this most recent information on the pupil and its reactions and thereby encourage other practitioners to intermittently measure the pupil with a portable instrument. Hopefully the following chapters will provide the framework to elevate this long-held interest in the pupil from just one of casual observation to an understanding that can benefit patients.

Chapter

1

Early History of the Pupil

The radiation diffuses from the psychic spirit that emerges from the brain to the pupil through the two hollow nerves that pass from the brain to the pupil. From there it spreads out in the air to visible objects so as to be an organ of the viewer.

(Qusta ibn Luqa, *Book on the Causes of the Difference in Perspectives*)

1.1 Ancient Greek and Roman Thoughts about the Pupil

Prehistoric societies would have readily learned the importance of the inner black circle (pupil) of the eye. Any obstruction to the passage of light through the pupil would block vision. Simply lowering the eyelid to cover the pupil obstructs vision, a fact the first humans would readily discover. Because of the vital importance of vision to survival in these early societies, preservation of the pupil and the apparatus of vision would have been paramount to survival. Little wonder therefore that the two concentric circles, the iris and the pupil, became one of the earliest icons of human societies, eventually to be replicated in all societies in their visual arts and religious symbols.

The mechanisms involved in vision have perplexed scholars for over 3,000 years. Hippocrates (460–370 BCE) mentions the pupil briefly and observed that it was a colorless, transparent liquid. He stated that it was only black because it was situated in the depths of the eye and surrounded by dark membranes. Over time, the ancient Greek philosophers developed conflicting ideas about vision and the function of the pupil. Two schools of thought emerged: the extramission theory and the intromission theory.

Plato (428–348 BCE) thought vision involved a vital energy that originated within the eye and passed through the pupil to the object in view. This energy or force was then combined with a visual ray emanating from the object and the combined force was then redirected into the eye where the image was formed and transmitted to the brain. This was the extramission theory that has persisted in one form or another even up to the present day. Plato was not the first to describe the extramission theory, but he promoted it, and it is often referred to after the Renaissance as the Neo-Platonism theory of vision.

Aristotle (384–322 BCE) drew upon the Hippocratic doctrine because he stated that the pupil was water (liquid) and furthermore it was in this liquid where the image was formed. His idea was that the viewed object sent out invisible rays and these rays reformed the object inside the pupil. This was the intromission theory. Aristotle's idea followed the well-known observation that a reflected image can be observed when one looks (carefully) at the pupil of another person. To Aristotle, this image in the water of the pupil was transmitted by the blood to the heart where perception took place. This intromission theory promoted by Aristotle rejected any rays coming out of the eye through the pupil, but instead noted that light passed into the eye. The actual image-forming portion of the eye was not known to the Greek or Roman thinkers, but both Aristotle and Plato thought that the image was formed within the pupil or just behind it in the crystalline lens.

Over 500 years later, Galen of Pergamon (129–216 CE) (Figure 1.1) was taught early in his career by Greek physicians founded in the cult of Asclepius, a society without a firm scientific foundation. During his life, Rome had emerged as the dominant society and his wealthy patrons were high-ranking Roman citizens, even the popular emperor Marcus Aurelius. Although he was a skilled theorist, many of his contributions were based on his own tireless observations. His early papers were the first ones to document life (i.e., movement) in the pupil. Galen thought that nature did nothing without a purpose and he saw marvelous workings in the human eye. Galen was a strong proponent of the

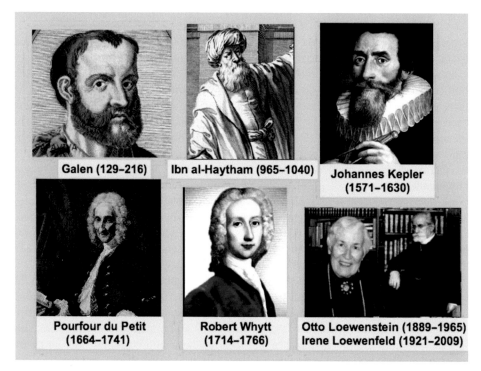

Figure 1.1 Prominent scientists who studied the pupil and pupil reactivity. Galen: Wellcome Library, London. Public Domain Mark, Reference 3349i. Ibn al-Haytham: Wikimedia Commons. Creative Commons CC0 License. Creative Commons Attribution-ShareAlike 4.0 International License. Johannes Kepler: Wellcome Library, London. Line engraving by N. Dietz. Public Domain Mark. Reference 4989i. Pourfour du Petit: Wellcome Library, London. Photogravure by I. Schutzenberger after J. Restout, 1737. License: Public Domain Mark. Robert Whytt: Wellcome Library, London. Available for reproduction under Creative Commons Attribution CC BY 4.0. Loewenfeld image: License Number: 5603830631563 from Wolters Kluwer Health, Inc. Lowenstein Image: License Number: 5614231355848 from Wolters Kluwer Health, Inc.

extramission theory and used his ideas to formulate diagnostic tests for visual acuity in preparation for cataract surgery (23).

Galen observed that if he blocked the light from entering one eye, it produced a dilation (widening) in the opposite pupil. His idea was that by blocking the vital spirits with an obstruction over one eye, they were prohibited from passing through that pupil, so they were then directed into the other side, i.e., the opposite pupil. With one side blocked from light, the spirits which would normally be directed through both eyes were now directed only into one eye, producing a more dilated pupil. He also thought that by closing one eye, this directed twice the amount of "pneuma" into only one eye and this improved the vision in the open eye.

Galen made the first true observations of pupillary activity, but his theory was erroneous and could not hold up to careful examination, even by his contemporaries who practiced medicine during his time. Pneuma, for example, was not supposed to be a substance at all . . . in other words, Galen's own description of pneuma that passed into the iris to inflate it and make it dilate was not matter at all because it was only a spirit. This pneuma was supposed to escape from the eye, then meet the object in view, and then return to the eye again and produce the image within the lens. From there, it was transported back to the lateral ventricle where perception took place.

But Galen describes the iris as inflating by an infusion of some substance like air or fluid, and in fact Galen claims to have demonstrated that the pupil could be made to dilate by injecting air or fluid into the anterior chamber of the eye. So, with Galen we have the first discovery, but also the first inconsistent and erroneous conclusion about how the pupil works. This uneasy balance between an observation and the explanation of why it occurs will be a consistent theme as we wind our way through this historical account of pupillary physiology.

Galen's discussion of the pupil was a practical one and directed toward the question of when (and if) to operate on a patient with a dense cataract. Removal of a cataract would only be beneficial if the visual apparatus behind the pupil was functionally intact. If a cataract was removed, the patient might still be blind if disease was also present behind the cataract. Thompson states (23) that Galen's test was to observe the good eye while blocking light intermittently to the diseased eye (the one contemplating extraction). With an intact posterior portion of the eye, the good eye should then intermittently constrict and dilate. Failing that sign, Galen would refuse to operate. As we further develop the story of the pupil, we will realize that Galen's test was valid, but his reasoning was faulty.

Galen's influence extended into the Renaissance. Paolo Veronese Caliari (1528–1588) created "The Creation of Eve" that can be viewed in the Art Institute of Chicago (Figure 1.2). The painting might be interpreted according to Galenic idea of vital energy emerging through the pupil. In the painting, the Lord covers one of Eve's eyes and observes the other eye. Galen had speculated that the opposite eye dilated because the vital energy that normally emanated through both eyes was now constrained to be released through only one eye. With this test, the Creator would confirm intact vision for Eve. Of course, the painting has many interpretations (24, 25).

Today, the science of ophthalmology is firmly in the intromission camp, but public opinion continues to be fascinated and wants to believe that there is an inner light that shines out through the pupil into three-dimensional space and illuminates objects in view. Science fiction movies commonly show creatures with light and laser beams emanating from the eyes that exert special powers on their intended targets. Is there

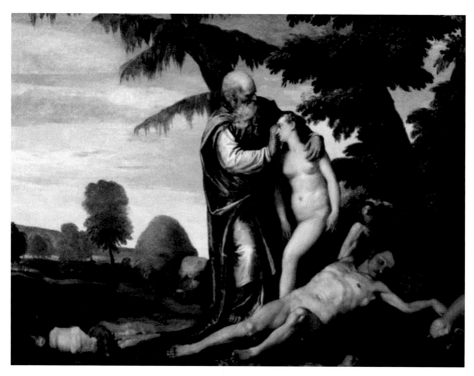

Figure 1.2 Paolo Venonese Caliari, *The Creation of Eve*, 1565–1575. The Art Institute of Chicago. The painting has many interpretations, but some authorities suggest that the Lord is testing for the presence of the light reflex. Image is made available under Creative Commons Zero designation from the Art Institute of Chicago CCO Public Domain Designation.

a role for the extramission theory in our modern construct of vision? It is now known that vision is not simply the processing of the retinal image by the visual cortex, a process that is well known to the perceptual sciences. But the inner light directs the pupil to focus a small area of the world view onto the fovea (see discussion in Chapter 2). The mobile eye is therefore crucial to our visual process and has its foundation in the works of scholars dating back several hundred years.

1.2 Arabic Scholars Advance the Science of Optics

With the fall of Rome, Western society slowly drifted into the Dark Ages, and Galen's work was nearly forgotten. The pupil was initially misunderstood by the early Arabic scholars (Figure 1.3) taking the Hippocratic idea that the pupil was a dark membrane inside the eye containing clear liquid.

Fortunately, Islamic medicine translated the works of the Greek physicians into Arabic, leading to the next major developments in our understanding of the pupil. Starting in the ninth century, several Arabic scholars such as Avicenna, Alhazen, Rhazes, and al-Kindi borrowed upon the optical treatises of Euclid, a Greek mathematician who lived in the third century BCE. They confirmed Euclid's theories that light travels in straight lines, but could not agree that light was emitted from within the eye.

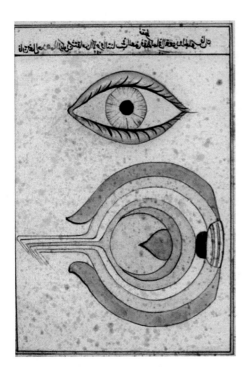

Figure 1.3 Early ninth-century Arabic illustration of the eye anatomy. Artist unknown. Property of author.

The Arabic scholars correctly thought that light enters the pupil and forms an image within the eye that is transferred to the brain for interpretation. Arabic scholars studied the works of Galen carefully, but they did not read his work as the final authority. Consequently, Islamic physicians made important original contributions to pupillary physiology.

Abu Bakr Muhammad Ibn Zakariya al-Razi, known as Rhazes (864–925 CE), is usually credited with being the first physician to note that light constricted the pupil. Rhazes, considered by some to be one of the greatest medical clinicians of all time, practiced in Baghdad and wrote extensively on many topics ranging from music to philosophy. He was the first to describe smallpox and differentiate that disease from measles. Although Rhazes described the light reflex, he continued the error that image formation occurred on the lens (or within the vitreous glassy humor), an error that was not corrected until the seventeenth century.

In retrospect, we know that Galen was really observing the effect of light on pupil diameter in the opposite eye (consensual reflex). Unfortunately, his adherence to the idea of vital spirits coming out of the eye prevented him from recognizing the fact that an increase in ambient light constricted the pupil. Today, we refer to this phenomenon simply as the light reflex, one of the most valuable clinical signs in the physical examination. In later chapters, we will return to the light reflex and explain why it is so important to clinical medicine. For now, however, it is only necessary to explain that Rhazes described the reflex, but was unable to explain why or how it occurred.

The observation by Rhazes significantly simplified the cumbersome test that Galen used to establish a functional retina and optic nerve behind a diseased lens. Rhazes and others observed that it was only necessary to observe the presence or absence of a light reflex in the diseased eye. Without the presence of a light reflex, there would be no point in removing a cataract because the clinical examination would indicate disease behind the lens. There are exceptions to this rule in patients who have tonic pupils and oculomotor nerve deficits that will be discussed in Chapter 5.

The optical treatises of Ibn al-Haytham (latinized as Alhazen, 965–1040 CE) became the initial source of information on how light is transmitted through the eye to produce an image. Alhazen was an Arabic philosopher who lived in the eleventh century. His interests were varied, but his legacy is due chiefly to his book entitled *Book of Optics*, written while he was sentenced to house arrest from 1011 to 1021. Alhazen was placed under house arrest because he thought he could dam the Nile River at Aswan. The Fatimid Caliph of Egypt (Al-Hakim bi-AmrAllah) commissioned him to achieve this feat, which with the engineering methods available in the eleventh century was soon discovered to be impossible. The Caliph was an intolerant ruler who severely punished his subordinates who were unable to fulfill their missions. To avoid being put to death, Alhazen feigned madness and was placed under house arrest where he had time to think about the nature of light and optics. During this time, he discovered basic principles of the camera obscura.

In the fourth century BCE, Aristotle had observed that, during a partial eclipse of the sun, crescent images were projected on the ground as the sunlight passed through a tree canopy (Figure 1.4). But Aristotle was not aware that light traveled in straight lines, so he was not able to envision the concept of the pin-hole camera. As previously discussed, Aristotle thought the visual image was captured by the lens and transmitted to the heart, where the image was processed. Although the Islamic scholars were familiar with Greek and Roman science, it is unlikely that the discovery of the camera obscura by Alhazen was influenced by Aristotle.

During the long hours that he spent under house arrest, Alhazen had time to contemplate the nature of light and develop his optical theories. The Caliph's edict thus eventually led to a book that has been ranked as one of the most influential books of all time relating to vision and optical theory. Alhazen observed the effect of light passing through small apertures. His famous experiment revealed that the passage of light through small holes (pupils) will project a reversed and inverted image on a screen. He reiterated Euclid's theories that light traveled in straight lines and then described the effect of lenses, mirrors, and prisms on the path of light rays. He successfully projected an

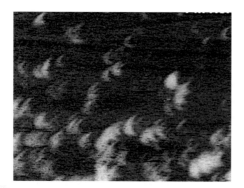

Figure 1.4 Images on the pavement below a tree canopy during a partial eclipse of the sun on October 23, 2014. Photograph by author.

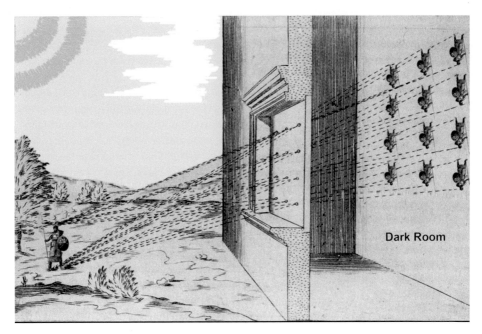

Figure 1.5 Alhazen illustrates the principles of inverted and reversed images through multiple holes into a dark room. Original drawing by Ping Hill, research assistance UCSF.

image through multiple holes onto a screen in a dark room and with these experiments he formulated the basic principle of the camera obscura (Figure 1.5). His invention initiated the scientific study of image formation that today accounts for nearly 2 trillion photographs taken annually.

Alhazen used his optical theories to explain vision by comparing the eye to the camera obscura. Thus, the pinhole became the pupil, and the interior of the eye became the screen upon which the image was projected. Although he erred in believing the lens was the structure on which the image was projected, he did hint that the retina might also have a role in image formation. Alhazen was puzzled as to how an inverted image in the eye could be transformed into an upright image by the mind. He concluded that the mind was able to interpret the image in the correct orientation, an idea that is surprisingly modern. For example, we now know that it is possible to adapt to glasses that invert the visual image.

Leonardo da Vinci (1452–1519) was familiar with the work of Alhazen and wrote several manuscripts about the eye and designed simple experiments that demonstrated the value of the pupil in forming the visual image. His description of the following experiment demonstrates how the pupil inverts and reverses an image. The description of this experiment is copied into print by Donald S. Strong (20) directly from Manuscript D in the Bibliotheque Nationale, Paris.

> Look directly at a blank wall that is illuminated with ambient light. Close the left eye and pass a toothpick from right to left in front of the right eye. It should be about 2 inches in front of the eye as it passes from right to left. The image of the toothpick will show the

blurred toothpick image that appropriately moves from right to left and this occurs because the light rays are reflected off the toothpick and directed onto the left side of the retina where the brain has been programmed to recognize objects in the right field of view. So far, this is a simple exercise that is just common sense. We see objects to the right of us when they on the right side of us.

Now punch a small 1–1.5 mm hole in a black piece of paper and position the hole about 3 inches in front of your right eye. Look through the small pinhole with your right eye onto the blank illuminated wall. Keep the left eye closed. You will observe a small white blurred disc. Now continue looking at this blurred disc and pass the toothpick from right to left in the same manner as was done previously. Again, the toothpick should be approximately 2 inches in front of the eye, between the eye and the black paper. Quite to your amazement you will observe the toothpick to move across the blurred disc from left to right! Now move the toothpick from top to bottom. The toothpick will move from bottom to top! What is happening? The toothpick has placed a shadow on the light rays that have passed through the pinhole. As the toothpick passes from right to left, it first encounters and blocks the light rays that have passed from the left visual field. The brain interprets this as a blocked light ray arriving from the left and as it passes from right to left, the shadow gradually passes from left to right. Note that the toothpick is actually moving from right to left, but the brain perceives it as moving from left to right. The same inversion occurs when the toothpick is moved up and down. In this example, the pinhole is an artificial pupil. The experimenter's pupil has no effect because it is larger than the pinhole. However, when the card is removed, the real pupil of the subject acts just like the pinhole, inverting and transposing the real image onto the retina.

Leonardo da Vinci also promoted several erroneous theories concerning vision, one of them relating to a secondary inversion within the vitreous humor which then produced an upright image that was transmitted to the brain by the optic nerve. And he accepted the false idea originating with Roger Bacon (1220–1292 CE) that the visual rays were reflected from the eyelashes into the pupil. Nevertheless, the writings of Bacon and da Vinci were significant because they disseminated to the Western world the concept of the human eye as a camera obscura as originally described by Alhazen (26).

As a parenthetic note, eyes that are based on the principle of the camera obscura are not necessary for vision. Insects have compound eyes wherein millions of individual tiny lenses concentrate light on a single photoreceptor. For humans to have the same image-forming capacity by using a compound eye, the size of our heads would be three times the size of our thorax and abdomen combined. The mammalian camera obscura eye makes it possible for us to economize on bodily space and still have the wide range of visual perception that we enjoy. Darwin was known to have remarked that to rationalize an eye developing strictly though evolution was one of the most difficult barriers to the promotion of his theories. The earliest light-sensitive organs were simple flat sheets of photoreceptors that allowed the organism to detect day and night, sunlight, and shadow. From this simple beginning, several evolutionary pathways led to the development of diverse and complex eyes in different animal species. Trilobites, octopus, squid, birds, insects, bees, and worms all have rudimentary eyes. They are different from ours and have developed through different evolutionary pathways. Most evolutionary biologists admit that at least eight different types of eyes developed from the earliest form of vision that occurred during the Cambrian era. Vision allowed organisms to proliferate to an extent not known during prior epochs and presumably led to the rapid increase in biologic diversity at that time.

Returning to Alhazen, he had recognized that the pinhole camera would project a clear image if the pinhole was very small. The small size of the pinhole pupil eliminated stray light that caused a blurred image with a larger pupil. The problem with the small-hole pupil was that the image was very faint because only a small amount of light could be passed through it onto the screen. Enlarging the hole (pupil) allowed more light to enter, but it also blurred the image because of the effects of stray light that entered the aperture along the perimeter of the opening. Alhazen's contribution was to describe the eye as an optical instrument, but the modern view was not elaborated until 500 years later.

The blurred image of the camera obscura was demonstrated and emphasized by Johannes Kepler (1571–1630) whom many credit with providing the first accurate description of the optics of the human eye. His teacher, Tyco Brahe (1546–1601), had given Kepler the assignment of measuring the precise diameter of the moon in minutes of arc. Kepler's interest was not in vision, but rather in planetary orbits, the diameter of the moon, and similar astronomical projects. His tool was the camera obscura. He examined the optics of the camera obscura by suspending visual objects, such as a book, from the ceiling of his room and then passing strings from various points of the object through a small aperture onto a screen. The image points on the screen could be improved significantly by decreasing the diameter of the pupillary aperture, but in practical use it became apparent that small diameter apertures produced too faint an image to be seen. Kepler promoted the idea of a lens to project an inverted and precise concentrated image onto the retina.

By the eighteenth century, the use of lenses to concentrate light had been fully appreciated. The lens behind the anterior chamber would concentrate the light onto a focused image which was then transmitted to the visual cortex and underwent interpretation. What was still unknown was the role of the retina in capturing the image. The vitreous was not connected to the optic nerve and thus was unlikely to be the image-forming structure. The layer below the choroid, called the retina by Galen, was the source of the fibers that eventually passed to the brain through the optic nerves. By the start of the eighteenth century, the optics of vision consisting of light entering the pupil, focused by a lens on the retina, and then transmitted into the optic nerve had been described by several scientists, including Rene Descartes and Johannes Kepler.

1.3 Reflex Action and the Pupil

In the eighteenth century, a controversy arose that was difficult to explain by the traditional explanations of how pupil size was controlled by light. The landmark treatise by Robert Whytt (1714–1766; Figure 1.1; 27, 28) in 1751 summarizes the controversy and provides us with an insight into how scientists often must wait until other information is forthcoming to explain unique physiological phenomena. Whytt was a Scottish physician with an uncanny ability to correlate clinical findings with pathologic lesions in the brain. He appeared to be a frail, timid, and unassuming person, but he was a man of tremendous energy and capacity for work. He had a large family, practiced clinical medicine, and rose to prominent positions within academia. He was the personal physician to George III and spent endless hours in correspondence with the leading physiologists of his day. Whytt's interests were vast and his major contribution to our story was only a small portion of his 1751 treatise on the involuntary functions of the body. His observations of pupillary behaviors in this one paper allowed him an understanding of the pupil that exceeds what most graduating medical students know today.

Since the time of Francis Bacon, there had been several theories about the mechanism whereby light constricts the pupil. Most commonly it was proposed that the iris contained some sensitive structure that responded directly to light. The muscle that surrounded the pupillary margin had been identified in the seventeenth century and a separate dilator muscle had been implicated by Pourfour du Petit (Figure 1.1). The dilator muscle was not precisely identified until the late nineteenth century (29).

Whytt observed several patients with no light reflex and correlated their postmortem pathology with their progressive symptoms prior to death. He concluded that the optic nerve carried an impulse into the brain where a "sentient principle" returned a response to the eye through another nerve (oculomotor), ultimately producing a contraction of the muscle surrounding the pupillary margin. Whytt was the first investigator to establish that much of human subconscious behavior consists of reflex action, whereby a stimulus sends a message into the central nervous system. Within the brain, modulating influences are brought to bear on the stimulus and then a response is directed to an effector organ, either a muscle or a secretory organ such as the adrenal or salivary gland. Whytt's idea for this modulating influence was to hypothesize a sentient principle or a "soul" to direct and control reflex activity designed to protect the organism. For example, the pupillary light reflex was organized by the sentient principle to protect the sensitive retina from damage from bright light.

Whytt's ideas were not immune from controversy. Albrecht von Haller (1708–1777) was only one of the many scientists with whom he had major disagreements. Only the passage of time has shown that Whytt's conclusions were for the most part correct. Whytt's case studies were important because they demonstrated that the brain was in control of unconscious responses such as could be observed in the response of the pupil to light. Thus, muscles do not respond to external stimuli by themselves, but only through a mechanism involving a reflex through the central nervous system. Marshall Hall (1790–1857) eventually carried the study of reflex action into the spinal cord, where flexion reflexes were observed in frogs that had been decapitated and were totally flaccid until they were stimulated (30).

Also, during the eighteenth century, Abbé Gasparo Ferdinando Felice Fontana (1730–1805) had described the effects of opium on the pupil and noted the unusual pupillary effects of sleep that are discussed in Chapter 10 on the "light off" (LO) reflex. He confirmed earlier reports that near vision was accompanied by a constriction of the pupil, that the pupil dilated at the moment of death and then gradually constricted to its final midposition (3–5 mm) diameter, and confirmed that a sympathy existed between the two eyes so that light directed into one eye would produce a light reflex in the other eye (31).

1.4 Inhibition of the Pupillary Light Reflex

Although the Islamic scholars had described the pupillary light reflex and Robert Whytt observed that it was a reflex action through the brain, there were other reports dating from the early seventeenth century that were difficult to explain. One of the issues was an experiment conducted in 1704 by J. Mery, who reported that submerging a cat in water caused the pupils to dilate and become unresponsive to light (32). Mery thought that the cat lost its vital spirits under water because it was unable to breathe. Normally these spirits filled and expanded the iris when light was exposed to it, and the loss of spirits resulted in a shrinkage of the iris. Pupillary dilation occurred when the vital spirits were diminished during asphyxia. Translating from the French article, he wrote: "light does not act on the iris directly but allows the 'espirts animaux' to enter; in blind eyes the pupil does not contract. In cat under water no spirits can enter and thus the pupil dilated by elasticity of the iris."

Others repeated Mery's experiment and verified that the submerged animal had dilated pupils that did not react to light. Philippe de la Hire (1640–1718) was a French mathematician and astronomer who also had an interest in optics. In the seventeenth century, mathematicians had eclectic interests and de la Hire wrote treatises on geology, architecture, zoology, and physiology. He noticed that bright light constricted the pupil of cats, but, if they were frightened, light had no effect on the pupil. His 1709 communication to the French Academy of Sciences deals with how vision takes place. In this treatise, he describes some valuable observations about the pupil that ushered in new ideas (33).

> But though we are exposed to a pretty strong light, we do not always close the pupil when we are attentive to look upon any object. We can observe this in those animals, which can close and dilate the pupil in an extraordinary manner, such as cats; for when they are in a strong light and quiet, their pupil is almost quite shut; and if any extraordinary object, which rouses their attention, presents itself, we see them open it at once as much as they can. In this regard, the following observation is pretty common, and those who have made it have always observed the same thing. If you plunge the head of a living cat into water, the pupil immediately quite opens itself, though the animal is exposed to a very bright object. This animal being in a violent state, gives attention to all that surrounds it, which must also oblige it to keep its pupil very open, as I have observed already.

Whytt had his own theory to explain these observations, which was just as erroneous. Whytt's idea was that under water the light could not be properly focused on the retina because of refraction of light rays at the air/glass/water interfaces. While there is undoubtedly a change in direction of light rays as they enter the liquid phase, the change in light intensity would still be present even though not precisely focused.

Albrecht von Haller (1708–1777) had his own ideas. Haller denied the presence of muscles in the iris because he was unable to confirm that the iris was irritable, which he thought was an essential property of all muscles (34). Instead, Haller maintained that all iris movements were brought about by engorgement or lack of engorgement of the iris blood vessels; submersion in water altered the blood vessels.

These authors could not arrive at the proper explanation because an essential feature of mammalian physiology at that time was not appreciated. Inhibitory processes in the nervous system were not described until the nineteenth century. E. H. Weber and others had presented the concept of inhibition in 1845 with classical studies on the inhibitory control by the vagus on heart rate (35). Sherrington demonstrated inhibitory processes in the spinal cord in his classic papers from 1906 (36). Brock, Coombs, and Eccles elegantly demonstrated synaptic inhibition in the spinal cord by recording intracellular potentials within motoneurons (37). These reports confirmed that inhibition does not occur at the neuromuscular junction, but it is a central event. Several authors then studied the effect of inhibitory control over the EW nucleus, a subject that will be further discussed in

Chapter 10 (13, 38, 39). Modern theory includes the blending of light flux, near fixation, and the emotional state of the subject as contributing factors that determine the size and reactivity of the pupil (40).

1.5 Looking into the Pupil

> She pulls an ophthalmoscope out of her bag and looks into Lenin's pupils. Papilledema, both sides, she says. Another sign of raised pressure in the brain.
>
> (Abraham Verghese, *The Covenant of Water*)

Until the early nineteenth century, the pupil was simply a black hole in the middle of the iris because there was no method to look through the hole. There had been many theories about why the eye became luminous under certain conditions. Some thought that the fleeting luminosity was a phenomenon of phosphorescence. Others speculated that light was absorbed during the day and emitted at night, while others thought that it was the result of activity similar to a firefly or that it was electricity emitted by the retina.

Even into the eighteenth century, the idea was still prevalent that the bright eyes of animals at night represented the visual rays emanating from the eyes to illuminate visual targets, a theory that had persisted since the days of the Greeks and Romans. But because the eyes of dead animals showed the same brightness, it soon became apparent that the light was reflected from the back of the eye along the same path as the light source. Any attempt to look through the pupil into the back of the eye brought about the difficult problem of how to look into the pupil. The observer's pupils either had to be closely behind the light source, in which case the light source blocked the observer's view – or the observer's pupil had to be in front of the light source, in which case the illumination from the light source was blocked and the pupil was only a black void.

Primitive societies had already discovered a use for the illuminated pupil. The entrance of light into the pupil was used by early societies to hunt at night. Robert Knox, an Englishman who lived in Sri Lanka in the mid seventeenth century, describes how the native population used the pupils to hunt at night (41).

Knox writes the following lines:

> Before I make an end of my discourse of their beasts, it may be worthwhile to relate the ways they use to catch them; at which they are very crafty.
>
> For the catching of deer, or other wild beasts, they have this ingenious device: in dark moons when there are drizzling rains, they go about this design: they have a basket made with canes, somewhat like unto a funnel, in which they put a pot-sheard with fire in it, together with a certain wood which they have growing there, full of sap like pitch, and that will burn like a pitch-barrel. This being kindled in the potsherd flames, gives an exceeding light. They carry it upon their heads with the flame foremost; the basket hiding him that is under it, and those that come behind it. In their hands they carry three or four small bells, which they tingle as they go, that the noise of their steps should not be heard. Behind the man that carries the light, go men with bows and arrows; and so they go walking along the plains, and by the pond sides, where they think the deer will come out to feed; which, when they see the light, stand still and stare upon it, seeing only the light, and hearing nothing but the tingling of the bells.

> The eyes of the deer, or other cattle, first appear to them glistening like stars of light or diamonds; and by their long experience they will distinguish one beast from another by their eyes. All creatures, as deer, hares, elephants, bears etc. excepting only wild hogs, will stand still, wondering at this strange sight till the people come as near as they do desire, and so let fly their arrows upon them; and by this means they seldom go but they catch something.

The glistening stars and diamonds that Knox describes are very similar but not identical to the well-known red-eye reflex that is so annoying to portrait photographers today. Most vertebrates have a mirror behind the retina called the *tapetum lucidum*. This is a thin layer of highly reflective tissue that directs the light back onto the photoreceptors so that they are stimulated twice for each light ray. It is highly developed in nocturnal animals and enhances their ability to see in low-lighting conditions. Humans do not have this mirror behind the retina, so the light of the so-called "red reflex" is the redness of the vascular layer that lies in front of the photoreceptors. It is still a reflected image of the back of the eyeball, but is not as vivid and clear as the bright circular reflected light from the mirrors behind the retinas of nocturnal animals. Most fish have the same layer of reflective tissue as the larger mammals.

A Mughal artist has illustrated how "pit lamping" was carried out in India (Figure 1.6). It was necessary for the archer to stand very closely behind the light source because the retinal reflection from the animal's eyes is passed through the pupils directly back to the light source. A hunter standing toward the side of the light source would not observe the brilliant diamonds.

The light that is reflected through the pupils became the stimulus for the invention of an instrument that allowed a look through the pupil into the eyeball, the ophthalmoscope. The solution to the problem was solved when, in 1847, Charles Babbage (1791–1871), an English mathematician, inserted a diagonal mirror into a small tube and directed a light onto the mirror through a small hole in the side of the tube. The mirror had a small open area in the center through which the reflected light could pass from the retina of the subject, then into the pupil of the observer. Babbage received no encouragement from ophthalmologists at the time and the idea was not developed further (42).

Hermann von Helmholtz (1821–1894) perfected Babbage's instrument in 1869. Today, a thorough physical examination is considered incomplete unless the physician looks through the patient's pupils to view the retinal blood vessels and the optic disc. It is now more than 150 years since Hermann von Helmholtz's discovery of the ophthalmoscope in 1851 (43). He called it an Augenspiegel (eye mirror). The name 'ophthalmoscope' (eye-observer) did not come into common use until three years later. At the time, Helmholtz was only 29. He was a professor of physiology and wanted to demonstrate to his students why the pupil of the eye sometimes appeared black and at other times had a red color.

For several years after the invention of the ophthalmoscope, the public was deceived into believing that images would persist on the retina even after death and could be viewed and photographed by specialists who could look with a special instrument through the pupil. Murder victims would have the image of their assailant printed on their retinas and then this special technician could look through the pupil into the eye to discover the murderer (44). Several cases of murder were adjudicated in court based on alleged "optograms" of the retina image at the time of death. Optograms of the retina turned out to be a totally false notion because the photoreceptors that transmit the image depend on a regular supply of oxygenated blood.

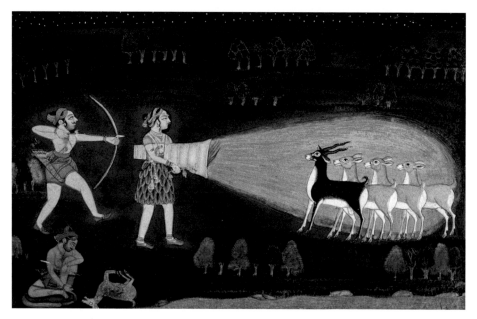

Figure 1.6 This painting from the Walters Art Museum, Baltimore, MD, illustrates how primitive societies used the reflection from the retina to hunt at night. The light reflected through the pupil was the target of the archer that was positioned behind the light source. Images are in the public domain, courtesy of the Walters Art Museum. *The Deer Hunt.* Artist: Jegdish Mittal, Hyderabad, India. Date: circa 1775. Gift of John and Berthe Ford.

1.6 The Pupil and the Autonomic Nervous System

A careful historical analysis reveals that various questions about pupillary behavior led to the discovery of the autonomic nervous system. Anatomy was a major discipline in the training of physicians in the early eighteenth century. Most of the prominent medical scientists had a firm foundation in the structures of the body. This new emphasis on teaching anatomy followed the gradual lifting of religious and political objections to human postmortem dissection. The publication of *De Human Corporis Fabrica* by Vesalius in 1654 was a major turning point because his atlas overturned the strict adherence to Galen's manuscripts that had by then been either translated from Arabic or from the original Greek texts into Latin. Vesalius uncovered several errors that Galen had made in describing human anatomy. We can partially excuse Galen because his errors were related to the fact that his dissections were made on non-human species. Human dissection was strictly prohibited in ancient Rome. Instead, Galen dissected cats, monkeys, dogs, rats, horses, cows, and even an elephant.

During the seventeenth century, the anatomy of the nervous system had been carefully and minutely detailed through the extensive work of Thomas Willis (1621–1675). In examining the manuscripts published by Willis, the neuroanatomists of the time must have been awed when they considered the meticulous attention that he paid to the anatomy of the brain and nerves.

Willis made a crucial mistake when he described the sympathetic nerves. His anatomy illustrated the origin of the sympathetic nerves in the brainstem. Over several years, a military surgeon by the name of François Ponfour du Petit (1664–1741) made observations that led to the designation of the autonomic nervous system as a separate entity from the brain. In 1703, Petit was recruited as a military physician in the armies of Louis XIV and traveled extensively during military campaigns in Spain and Gibraltar. He must have been a naturally curious individual because his careful examination of wounded soldiers led to a description of contralateral paralysis after extensive head wounds to one side of the skull. This alone would have secured du Petit a prominent position in the annals of neurology. However, he had other questions about anatomy that continued to puzzle him for several decades, which revolved around a peculiar syndrome that he had observed in 1713. A soldier who had a case of pulmonary disease was observed to have an unusual clinical syndrome involving the eye on the same side as the pulmonary abnormality – a droopy eyelid and a dull eye. Du Petit was curious about this patient because Willis and other anatomists would not have predicted any clinical abnormalities above the level of the pathology (the eye being more cephalad to the thorax) because the Willis anatomy showed that the innervation of the eye arose solely from the brain.

Luckily for the advancement of knowledge about the pupil, du Petit was not intimidated by the exhaustive work of Willis. Based on certain inconsistencies in the work of Willis, du Petit made the next major step in deciphering how pupil size and reactions are controlled. In doing so, his work led to the discovery of the sympathetic nervous system. He then carried out experiments on dogs that confirmed his earlier suspicion that the nerves in the neck and upper thorax controlled certain functional aspects of the eye, including the size of the pupil. His anatomical studies showed that these nerves arose from the spinal cord and traveled up the neck and innervated the eye from below (45). These findings revealed a major inconsistency in the current thinking about the innervation of the eye. If the nerves to the eye that produced these symptoms went up the neck from below, then the vital fluid must also flow in a direction opposite (retrograde) to what Willis had proposed. Willis, Vesalius, Galen, and all the anatomists prior to du Petit had shown the intercostal nerve, from which the eye was partially innervated, arose from cranial nerves 5 and 6, and therefore the vital spirits flowed from these nerves from the brain into the orbit in the normal (antegrade) forward fashion.

It took nearly 150 years before the significance of du Petit's findings was appreciated. Several prominent physiologists were involved in explaining his unusual observations. Claude Bernard (1831–1878) repeated and expanded on du Petit's experiments in the late nineteenth century, and Johann Fredrick Horner (1831–1886) described the clinical syndrome that bears his name in 1867. Today, the clinical signs of Horner's syndrome are known by all practicing physicians as a guide to detect interference with the sympathetic nervous system at specific sites within the central and peripheral nervous system.

Finally, du Petit's observation on the pupil was the beginning of our understanding of the secondary nervous system, the one that is referred to as the autonomic nervous system. Near the end of the nineteenth century, much of John N. Langley's (1852–1925) work on the autonomic nervous system, which won him the Nobel Prize in 1910, was performed on the pupil. H. K. Anderson first described the phenomenon of paradoxical pupillary dilation in 1903 (46). This is an unusual phenomenon that occurs when the nerve fibers to a particular end organ are interrupted. When this occurs, the body attempts to compensate by increasing the reactivity of the receptors that respond to the transmitters released by the nerve (47). It is a property of nearly all receptors in the peripheral and central nervous system and has been extensively studied by physiologists since its description by Anderson on the receptors of the dilator muscle of the iris. Several investigators, including Cannon and Rosenblueth (48), later studied the mechanisms involved in producing paradoxical dilation and their studies formed the basis for our understanding of denervation hypersensitivity (see discussion of Figure 13.2 in Chapter 13).

2

Anatomy of the Pupil

> He held a police-watch over the pain-pressed pilgrim. When the pilgrim tried to rest, he opened those same lids wide, with pitiless finger and thumb, and gazed deep through the pupil and the iris into the brain, into the heart, to search if vanity, or pride, or falsehood, in any of its subtlest forms was discoverable in the furthest recess of existence.
>
> (Charlotte Bronte, *Villette*)

Historical accounts relating to the pupil are based on a sound understanding of the anatomy of the orbit. Our understanding of the anatomy of the eye arose first in ancient Greece and Rome, when scholars dissected the eye carefully and named each layer by comparing it to some aspect of nature (Figure 2.1). The identifying features of the eye thus have their origins in two ancient languages, Greek and Latin, and the words derived from these languages have been used for several centuries.

The outermost covering of the eye is called the *sclera* from the ancient Greek work for hard, for example, and is the tough tunic of the eyeball. *Cornea* is the clear hard and firm projection of the sclera that covers the front part of the eye. The word derives from *cornua*, meaning like a horn, because the Greek anatomists compared the cornea to the horn of a sheep or ram. Below the cornea and sclera is the *uvea*, or grape (*uva* is Greek for grape) because without the sclera, the eye looks like a ripe grape. The uvea contains three parts. In front is the *iris*, named after the Roman goddess of the rainbow. Iris was the messenger between the Gods and man. It is the part of the eye that gives it color and forms the pupil by its free central margin. The word implies that the population of Greece and Rome had citizens with a variety of iris pigments. The *palpebral fissure* is the space between the upper and lower eyelids; this fissure ordinarily covers the upper portion of the circular iris. Palpebra is the Latin term for eyelid.

Next to the iris is the *ciliary body*, so named because of the fine threads (cilia) that connect it to the *crystalline lens*. *Cilia* in Latin means eyelash, so these threads were compared to the eyelash. The word crystalline relates to the similarity of the lens to ice, and the word lens comes from lentil because the lens is shaped like a lentil seed. The lens can also be translated in Latin as the *vitreous pica*, as *pica* means a bridge or stationary pillar, so the lens was thought of as a clear glass (vitreous) that was secured by the ciliary body in a stable position. Further back and around the side is the *choroid*, the third portion of the uvea. The name stems from the Greek word for the nutritive covering of the fertilized ovum. The ancient Greek thought was that the choroid provided nutrition to the retina. Below the choroid is the *retina*, from the word *rete*,

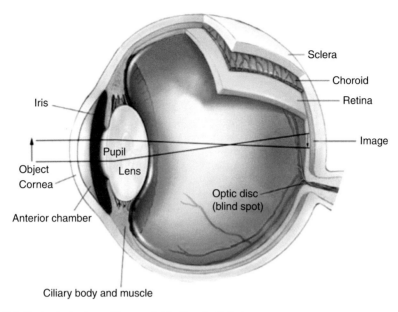

Figure 2.1 The basic structure of the eye. Public Domain, Getty Images.

meaning net. The retina is the photosensitive portion of the eye and can be compared to the film of a camera. Rod and cone photoreceptors send their signals to ganglion cells that comprise the major output cells of the retina. Some ganglion cells are intrinsically photosensitive and have been called intrinsically photosensitive retinal ganglion cells (ipRGCs) (49). These ganglion cells contain melanopsin and send projections to the suprachiasmatic nucleus as well as the pretectal region to initiate the pupillary light reflex. The ganglion cells leave the orbit via the optic nerve in an area that can be visualized through an ophthalmoscope, the optic disc. The *macula lutea* (yellow spot) is an area of increased vascularity around the *fovea centralis* (central pit). The fovea is the most sensitive portion of the retina. The vitreous is a mass of clear gelatinous material that lies behind the lens and in front of the retina. The name derives from the Latin work for glass.

Notably missing from these nature-derived anatomical terms is the word *pupil* because it is not an actual physical structure. The word derives from the Greek word *pupillae*, meaning orphan, or little child. "Pupil" therefore refers to the small, reflected image that one can see when looking (closely) into the pupil of another person.

The pupil is a mysterious portion of the human anatomy. It is a void, an emptiness. When we investigate the pupil from the outside, we see only a black hole. The pupil and the light-sensitive portions of the eye are part of the brain, but we are frustrated when we try to understand how the brain or how vision works by looking into the pupil. Even with an ophthalmoscope that allows us to see inside the eye, the view we obtain is unimpressive compared to what we know the eye performs for us. No wonder that the mystery of vision has always fascinated mankind and will continue to do so in the future. Like the character in Charlotte Bronte's novel, we expect to see the inner workings of the brain when we look through these black holes. Neither the black holes of outer space nor those of the brain can be analyzed by traditional scientific methods. They cannot be touched, weighed, chemically analyzed, smelled, vaporized, or heard. In the eye, this radiant energy is transformed into images that are coded into conscious sensations of three-dimensional space, but without the pupil this light would be just a diffuse blur on the back of the eye.

The pupil is a slightly eccentric circular opening from the anterior into the posterior chamber of the eye and is formed by the inner free edge of the iris. Its size can vary approximately fourfold by the activity of two groups of muscles that reside within the iris stroma. This wide range of movement makes it one of the most highly variable parameters that can be assessed by physicians. By contrast, for example, other common measures of autonomic activity such as heart rate and blood pressure rarely triple in magnitude, as is often the case with pupillary diameter.

The smooth muscles that control pupil size are unique. In contrast to other smooth muscles, the intrinsic muscles of the iris derive from the same ectodermal embryonic tissue that forms the brain and peripheral nervous system. The pupil changes in size because of the contraction of two sets of muscles that are embedded within the iris stroma, the *sphincter pupillae* and the *dilator pupillae*. The Greek physicians noticed that the pupil was very small at times and used the word *miosis* to describe that condition, *miosis* meaning shuteye. *Mydriasis*, also of ancient Greek derivation, means a widely dilated pupil.

The pupillary aperture is absent in the fetus, and it is another one of the miracles of nature that the membrane that covers the pupillary opening in the unborn child disintegrates within the first few weeks of life. Rarely this embryonic pupillary membrane persists and must be removed surgically. It should be mentioned that there are individuals who are born without pupils. The condition is an inborn error of development and is termed *aniridia* . . . in other words, these patients do not have an iris and thus there is no pupil in the traditional sense of the word. The limbus, or the junction of the cornea with the sclera, provides a substitute pupil in these patients. Because the diameter of the cornea is usually about 10 mm, these patients have a severe visual handicap and are unable to enter daylight environments without protective sunglasses. The 10 mm "pupil" is unable to focus properly, and consequently the patients are usually considered blind.

The two sets of muscles that control pupil size are oriented so that when activated, they oppose each other. The parasympathetic muscle, sometimes referred to as the pupillary sphincter, is a concentric band along the inner free margin of the iris that acts like a purse string to close the pupillary aperture. It is activated by muscarinic cholinergic fibers that reach it via the ciliary ganglion, in turn controlled by the Edinger–Westphal (EW) nucleus.

Frequent reference will be made in later chapters to the EW nucleus. The preganglionic neurons in the upper midbrain that initiate the pupillary light reflex were first described by Ludwig Edinger in 1885 (50) and later by C. F. O. Westphal in 1887 (51). These neurons occupy a separate area in the oculomotor nucleus of the third cranial nerve. This EW nucleus also contains neurons that innervate the ciliary muscle and change the shape of the lens. This reflex is part of the near reflex triad that includes convergence, lens accommodation, and pupillary constriction.

Today, it is known that the EW nucleus is divided into the preganglionic neurons that project to the ciliary ganglion (EWpg) and another group of cells that have been labeled the "centrally projecting EW neurons" (52, 53). This EWcp group of neurons is not involved in the pupillary reflexes. Throughout this book, the designation "EW" will refer to the EWpg neurons that control the size of the pupil. Recent electron micrographs and trans-synaptic labeling methods have observed that the neurons associated with pupillary constriction have many inhibitory contacts that are not observed in the lens-associated neurons (54). The importance of inhibitory control over the firing rate of the EW will be discussed in later chapters.

The sympathetic dilator muscle is innervated by the sympathetic nerves that originate in the upper thoracic spinal cord. This nerve synapses with the postganglionic nerve in the superior sympathetic ganglion. From there, it traverses a pathway into the orbit near the internal carotid artery and the cavernous sinus. Lesions of the nerve along this circuitous pathway can produce Horner's syndrome and often will present a diagnostic challenge to locate the pathological lesion. The sympathetic dilator muscle interdigitates with the sphincter muscle near the iris free margin and then fans out in a radial orientation toward the limbus junction of the iris and the sclera. Activation of this radially oriented muscle by the sympathetic nervous system pulls at the pupillary free margin and dilates the pupil (13).

As mentioned previously, the muscles of the iris are embryonically part of the brain. The ectodermal origin of the iris musculature is true for mammals, but is rare across the animal kingdom. The octopus, for example, has eyes that are very similar to the mammalian eye, but the muscles that control the octopus's pupil are entirely mesodermal in origin. As our story of the pupil unfolds, it will become apparent that this close association between the eye and the central nervous system presents a research tool that allows us to study what goes on inside the brain. Although Leonardo da Vinci repeated the idea that the pupil is the "window to the soul," his meaning was simply that a visual sensation must first enter the pupillary aperture before it could produce sensation. The understanding of how emotions and mental processing can alter pupil size and reactivity is a twentieth-century discovery.

Although the above paragraphs describe the pupil, it should be mentioned that the word "pupil" is used carelessly in our conversations and also in the world literature. For example, in his 1856 novel *The Man Who Laughs*, Victor Hugo writes: "The Duchess had a peculiarity, less rare than it is supposed. One of her eyes was blue and the other black. Her pupils were made for love and hate, for happiness and misery." Here, Hugo refers to a condition known as heterochromia and implies that the two pupils have different colors, when in fact the iris is the colored pigmented structure that surrounds the black pupil. When an author states that "the pupils widened," this usually means that the eyelids became more separated so that the entire iris becomes visible by the observer. Ordinarily, the upper eyelid covers a very small portion of the upper margin of the iris, and when this eyelid is raised, it is commonly stated that the pupils dilate. The actual size of the iris or the pupil does not change, but rather it appears to enlarge because of an optical illusion. Surprise, fear, anxiety, and pain all widen the orbital (palpebral) fissure and reveal the full iris circle. The pupil might also dilate slightly, but an observer from a distance cannot detect the small changes in the diameter of the pupil, especially in someone with dark eyes.

It is often stated that Chinese merchants could ascertain a customer's penchant for their products by observing their pupils. If this is true, it is an art that has never been developed in Western societies and today is probably a lost art even in China. As will be discussed in a subsequent chapter, the pupillary dilation that occurs during arousal is only about 1 mm (usually less), and it would take an astute observer to notice this change. It is far more likely that the iris appears to dilate through the effect of widening of the palpebral fissure, allowing the full circle of the iris to be visible. Of course, it is possible that the pupil could be assessed in this situation, but the merchant's lighting fixtures would have to be carefully arranged so that the pupil could be visualized.

Chapter 3

Physiology of the Pupil

And the pupil having received the objects, by means of the light, immediately refers them and transmits them to the intellect.

(Leonardo da Vinci, *The Notebooks of Leonardo da Vinci*)

The light reflex pathway originates with photon capture in the retina and elicits the light reflex through the pathway into the olivary pretectal nucleus as shown in Figure 3.1. The olivary pretectal nucleus activates the EW nucleus, which then projects to the ciliary ganglion. As mentioned in the previous chapter, the preganglionic pupilloconstrictor (EW) neurons have both excitatory and inhibitory afferent connections. The intrinsic photosensitive retinal ganglion cells (ipRGCs) are activated by light and provide the primary afferent input that generates the pupillary light reflex. These cells contain melanopsin, which responds to short wavelengths, but they also receive input from the rods and cones, activated by longer wavelengths. Although there may be some differences in the extent of the reflex depending on the wavelength of the simulating light, for the purpose of our discussion, the reflex is generated with commercial pupillometers using white light.

Modern techniques of recording from neurons in the brain have elegantly illustrated how inhibition at the EW nucleus can alter pupil size (Figure 3.2). These recordings by Sillito and Zbrozyna (55) show the rapid firing rate of the EW neurons during anesthesia. Addition of light produces only a small increase in their firing rate, but an arousal stimulus totally inhibits their activity, and the pupil dilates as the sphincter relaxes. The inhibition outlasts the stimulus. As is shown in Figure 3.2, a light stimulus, shown by the lines below the spikes from the neuron, is briefly ineffective in constricting the pupil for several seconds after the stimulus. Presumably this occurs because of the strong post-illumination inhibitory influence on the nucleus. These neuronal recordings may explain why the light reflex is briefly depressed during anesthesia following an intense noxious stimulus (18). The recordings by Sillito and Zbrozyna were taken from chloralose-anesthetized cats, but the constricted pupil is also observed during anesthesia in humans with commonly used agents (55). Elegant studies by Loewenfeld over 60 years ago demonstrated that intense nociception during anesthesia can depress the pupillary light reflex through inhibition of the EW nucleus (13). The same effect occurs in humans during surgical anesthesia when an intense stimulus dilates the pupil (56, 57).

The excitatory light pathway passes from one eye through the olivary pretectal nucleus into both sides of the EW nucleus. The reflex is therefore consensual in humans, meaning that a stimulus in one eye will contract both pupils. Some investigators have observed that the non-simulated eye has a very slightly decreased reflex compared to the stimulated eye. Neurotransmitters for this afferent pathway into the EW nucleus are

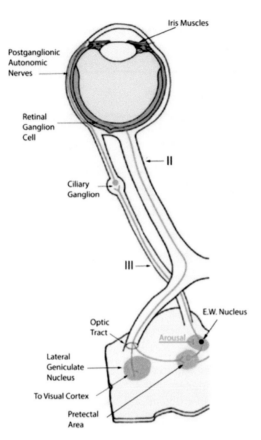

Iris Muscles

Postganglionic
Autonomic
Nerves

Retinal
Ganglion
Cell

II

Ciliary
Ganglion

III

E.W. Nucleus

Optic
Tract

Arousal

Lateral
Geniculate
Nucleus

To Visual Cortex

Pretectal
Area

Figure 3.1 The light reflex is a brain stem reflex that is modified by cortical and spinal afferent pathways. E.W. nucleus – Edinger Westphal nucleus; II – Optic nerve; III – Third cranial nerve, oculomotor. Figure drawn for publication by Ping Hill, Research Intern, University of California, San Francisco.

unknown, but it is known that NMDA receptor blocking agents such as ketamine and nitrous oxide depress the pupillary light reflex, so a glutamate neurotransmission is assumed at some synaptic junction (58). The retina and the pretectal nucleus have "light on" and "light off" (LO) responses that contribute to the shape of the reflex. Additional contributions to the waveform of the light reflex are made by the sympathetically innervated dilator muscle.

The portable instruments use light stimulation intensities and durations that approximate the pen-light examination of a flash in each eye to observe pupillary constriction and dilation. More details on the stimulus duration and illumination levels are discussed in Chapter 6 and in the Glossary. As described in Chapter 2, the size of the pupil is controlled by two sets of smooth muscle that are located within the iris. As with many other autonomic systems, these two muscles antagonize each other in their effect on pupil size, though relaxation of the sphincter and tension in the radial muscles are sometimes simultaneous events that will produce a larger effect than either muscle acting alone.

The pupillary responses to light depend on the circumstances under which the measurements are taken. The amplitude of the reflex, the waveform shape, and latency are dependent on the intensity of the light, the duration of the stimulus, and the location

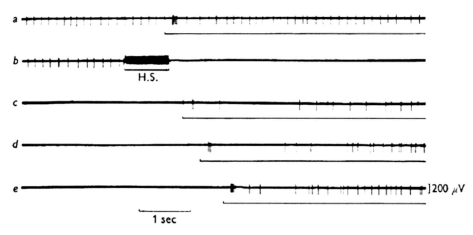

Figure 3.2 These recordings from the EW nucleus from chloralose-anesthetized cats reveal the characteristics of the EW nucleus neurons during light and noxious stimulation. The pupils are constricted because of the anesthetic. A light stimulus, shown by the line under each recording, has only a very slight stimulating effect on the firing rate of the neurons. In b, a noxious electrical stimulus was delivered and the neurons are inhibited. There is a prolonged pause in the firing rate, but a light stimulus will gradually reestablish the constricted pupil size and the spontaneous EW activity. Permission for reproduction of image from John Wiley & Sons, License Number: 5593181429109.

on the retina where the light is directed. These features can be altered with some commercially available portable infrared pupillometers, but for many clinical indications, the stimulus parameters are set for each instrument and would not be altered during repeated examinations.

Each investigator has unique instruments and a separate experimental design. For example, stimulating with a short wavelength stimulus of blue light will produce an atypical post illumination pupillary response (PIPR) (59, 60). This response is generated by the intrinsically photosensitive melanopsin containing retinal ganglion cells that respond to blue light. When stimulated with a selective light within the band of 479 nanometers, the pupil exhibits this atypical response at "light off." The same response is not prevalent with longer wavelength or white-light stimulations. At illumination levels that are used with portable instruments, there is no difference in the pupillary response waveform when the stimulus is a white light source compared to a light source with selective removal of the blue wavelengths that activate the melatonin sensitive photoreceptors (ipRGCs) (61). The study of PIPR may have relevance to the diagnosis of certain diseases of the retina. The portable pupillometers that are used clinically stimulate the retina with white light on each measurement and do not produce a PIPR. Although light stimuli with different waveform characteristics might become important to incorporate into portable instruments, at this time it is a unique form of simulation for the neuro-ophthalmologists using office-based pupillometers.

It is commonly thought that the pupil has basically two reflexes, the light reflex and reflex dilation. But the pupil is connected to the brain, the most complex organ in the body. This therefore makes the pupil likewise complicated. Irene Loewenfeld's book on the pupil is 1,500 pages long, with more than 14,000 references, and thousands of publications postdate the last issue of her book from 1999. A lengthy treatise could be

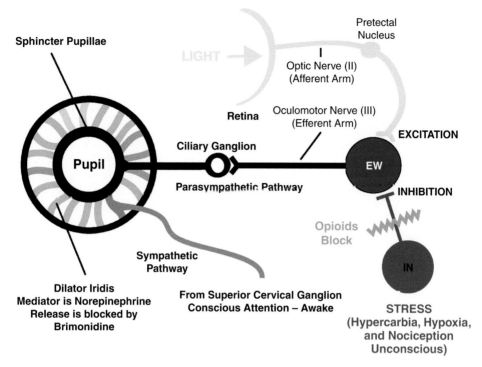

Figure 3.3 Control of pupil size is illustrated here. Permission granted to reproduce this image from Wolters Kluwer Health, Inc. License Number: 5591960791895.

written on the physiology of the pupil. In addition to the light on reflex, there is the light off (LO) reflex and pupillary unrest in ambient light (PUAL). These topics will be discussed in later chapters. More extensive discussions on pupillary physiology can be found in reviews on the subject (62, 63).

Cortical brain structures can produce subtle changes in pupil size and reactivity (64–66). These cortical pathways are incompletely described, but presumably are directed into the midbrain centers that control pupil size and reactivity (Figure 3.3). Examples that use these methods to activate cortical influences on the pupil include subtracting serial numbers, multiplication tasks, the idea of brightness, forced conversations, discrimination of different pitch, recall of digits, and provocations of threat. In these studies, the pupil size changes are 0.5 mm or less and require strict attention to ambient lighting and stable recording conditions. Accurate pupillometric measurement is essential because repeating a study would be difficult unless attention to recording details is adhered to. Standards of pupillometry measurements have been published (67, 68). Many of these psychophysiological studies use eye goggles, desk top pupillometers, high-frequency recordings, and averaging techniques. Portable infrared pupillometry may have a role in retrieving useful data from these types of studies (69). This research might be used in the future by psychologists and psychiatrists to manage therapy. Much of this work has been summarized from articles by Stuart Steinhauer (63–66) and by a recent book on the topic (70).

Pharmacology of the Pupil

> One child ate four ripe berries of the belladonna, another ate six. Both one and the other were guilty of extravagancies which astonished the mother; their pupils were dilated; their countenances no longer remained the same; they had a cheerful delirium, accompanied with fever. They were purple and their pulse hurried.
>
> (Isaac Disraeli, *Curiosities of Literature*, Volume 2, Part 4, 1835)

Approximately 400 years ago, nerves were thought to be similar to a series of long tubes (71). It was believed that a vital spirit passed through these tubes to activate muscles. When the spirit arrived at the muscle, it inflated the muscle, initiating movement. Vision was also made possible by this spirit coming through the pupil and striking an object to illuminate it for the mind to see. Galen used this idea to explain why the opposite pupil gets larger when one eye is covered. One difficulty with this explanation of nervous transmission was that muscles do not become inflated when the nerve activates them. This was revealed in a simple experiment performed in the seventeenth century wherein the arm of a muscular subject was placed under water. As the subject flexed his muscles, there was no change in the water level, indicating that the mass of muscle did not increase when the nervous spirits entered it and made it contract (72).

The idea that the brain was a complicated mesh of nerve networks that left the central nervous system in the form of long nerves was only discovered within the past 150 years. Several anatomists had detected under light microscopy that most central neurons were not actually connected, but a gap was present between neurons. Furthermore, there was a distinct apparatus at the junction of one nerve with the next one. Sir Charles Sherrington called this junction the "synapse," a word that is now over 100 years old. The original word synapse was coined by Sherrington in 1906 after the Greek work signifying "connect" (36). Until approximately 100 years ago, it was thought that these synaptic junctions were simply areas where the electrical impulse of one nerve cell transferred its electrical impulse to the next nerve cell. By 1915, it had been discovered that instead of a vital spirit moving down the nerves, a progressive wave of ionic movements across the membrane (specifically sodium ions) accounted for a form of electricity that moved along the nerve fibers, both within the brain and along peripheral nerves.

The pupil played a large role in developing our current theories of neurochemical transmission between neurons and between neurons and muscles. This came about largely because the receptors that respond to these chemicals can be activated by topical application of drugs onto the surface of the cornea. The changes in the pupillary reactions brought about by topical applications of drugs can be readily observed with infrared pupillometry.

Study of the pupil led to the idea of chemical transmission between nerves. Thomas R. Elliott was a young graduate student who studied under the tutorship of the prominent scientist John N. Langley. In 1904, Elliott proposed the novel idea that nerves were communicating with each other and with muscles by releasing a chemical into the synaptic cleft. This chemical then acted on the adjacent nerve or muscle to alter its excitability. Of course, the idea was soundly rejected immediately; even Elliott himself began to doubt the theory. In Elliott's view, the message from one nerve to another was transmitted by specific chemicals and not by any form of electrical process. His idea came to him through his studies on the pupil in the following manner: electrical activation of the sympathetic nerve in the neck would dilate the pupil. This was known since the time of Claude Bernard. Topical adrenalin placed on the surface of the eye would also dilate the pupil of the cat. How did adrenalin dilate the pupil? Was adrenalin inciting the nerve into action? Elliott reasoned that if he cut the nerve, then adrenalin should have no effect on the pupil if the nerve was required for its pupil dilating effect. To his surprise, the dilating effect of adrenalin became even more pronounced after cutting the nerve. His remarkable conclusion was published in a very short article in the Proceedings of the Physiological Society of London in 1905: "Adrenalin might be the chemical stimulant liberated on each occasion when the impulse arrives at the periphery" (73). This was the beginning of our ideas about neurochemical transmission in the central and peripheral nervous system. Although Elliott had the right interpretation, it took another 17 years until Elliott's theory became widely accepted. His mentor, John N. Langley, gave little encouragement to the young graduate student and within a few years, Elliott had left academia and spent the remainder of his career as a clinician. In 1921, Otto Loewi demonstrated the proof of chemical transmission that was initially suggested by Elliott. Loewi's classic studies were performed on the isolated hearts of frogs and demonstrated the vagal cholinergic inhibition of heart rate (74). Today, we are aware that central neurons can also communicate via simple electrical transmission without a neurotransmitter mediator.

4.1 Topical Application of Drugs

The autonomic receptors on the iris muscles can be activated by topical applications of drugs onto the corneal surface. So, it is not surprising that the early pharmacologists used the pupil to gain an understanding of how drugs produced their effects on the body. We are all aware of the importance of placing eye drops onto the surface of the eye during a visit to the ophthalmologist. This maneuver simply floods the muscle receptors in the eye with a chemical so that it cannot respond to its natural neurotransmitter. The historical development of our ideas about topical medication of the eye is closely intertwined with the discovery of how nerve cells in the brain and the peripheral nervous system communicate with each other. Several interesting stories are written relating to how these drugs were discovered and the role of the pupil in understanding how they produce their biologic effect. They often involve adventure, indigenous medicine, exploration, primitive herbal medicines, astute clinicians, and self-experimentation. An experiment with a newly discovered plant formulation was relatively easy in the nineteenth century, a time when many of the key advances were made in understanding how the brain and drugs interact. One hundred and fifty years ago, the key ingredients to perform a scientific experiment on the pupil were an extract of the agent and a willing subject who would allow these rudimentary preparations to be topically applied onto their corneas. Lacking these ingredients, we might not have had the extensive understanding that we have today about the interaction of plants and the human body. Much of our understanding of how chemical transmission takes place and how various drugs interact with this process was obtained by studying the pupil. The first section of this chapter discusses various topical agents that can alter pupil size.

4.1.1 Cocaine

A study of the pupillary effects of cocaine provided one of the major breakthroughs in our understanding of how the nervous system is altered by drugs. Cocaine is the active ingredient in the plant *Erythroxylon coca* that is indigenous to the eastern slope of the Andes in South America. When the Spanish explorers arrived, they took note of the reverence that the local population had for this plant. Although it was originally used as a central stimulant primarily by the Inca rulers, by the time the Spanish arrived in the sixteenth century, nearly all of the local inhabitants were using the plant as a mood enhancer, very similar to the use of coffee in our society. The coca leaves were brought back to Europe as early as the late sixteenth century, but it was not until the mid nineteenth century that the primary active ingredient, cocaine, was isolated and studied as an independent agent. Eventually it was learned that coca leaves contain up to 20 other alkaloids in addition to cocaine, so chewing the leaves is not the same as ingesting cocaine.

Cocaine was isolated from the indigenous South American shrub *Erythroxylon coca* in 1860. Twenty-eight years later, a young Austrian ophthalmologist, Carl Koller, dropped a solution of cocaine onto the eye and demonstrated its ability to block sensation, thus providing for painless surgery on the anterior chamber of the eye. The study and alteration of the cocaine molecule eventually led to the development of newer and safer local anesthetics, ushering in the entire specialty of regional anesthesia. Parenthetically, Koller also noted that topical cocaine dilated the pupil.

As is often the case in this narrative, the mydriatic effect of cocaine was essentially a side effect, but it remains as one of the few uses of cocaine in contemporary medical practice, and the understanding of its pupil-dilating effect led to significant advancements in our understanding of neurochemical transmission. The pupil-dilating effect of cocaine puzzled the early investigators who thought it might be related to the increase in heart rate and blood pressure often seen after the systemic administration of the drug. Eventually, pharmacologists discovered that cocaine possessed an interesting property that enhanced the effect of norepinephrine after it was released from the nerve ending. It seems that most of the released norepinephrine is taken back into the same nerve terminal from which it was released and that this action is the primary one that terminates the effect of norepinephrine on the dilator muscle. Cocaine has the property of preventing this reuptake. This effect enhances the effect of norepinephrine on the muscle, and the pupil dilates. Cocaine has therefore found a role in the diagnosis of Horner's syndrome. The patient with Horner's syndrome has very little or no norepinephrine in the sympathetic nerves innervating the dilator muscle, so topical application of cocaine will not dilate the Horner's pupil. Newer agents such as apraclonidine are now used that have advantages over cocaine in the diagnosis of Horner's syndrome. A brief discussion of Horner's syndrome as it relates to anesthetics and opioids will be included in the next chapter.

4.1.2 Atropine and Scopolamine

Atropine and scopolamine are among the oldest drugs known to mankind. Their use dates back as far as 3000 BCE. The gradual realization that a dilated and nonreactive pupil was associated with use of these drugs arose prior to the rise of modern medicine. Loewenfeld states that Galen used nightshade (a plant containing scopolamine) to dilate the pupils prior to cataract extraction. Several hallucinogenic plants contain atropine and scopolamine, and observations of shamans and witch doctors throughout the centuries under the influence of these drugs would report dilated pupils. However, whether that was due to the agents themselves and not to the general state of central nervous system excitement was difficult to analyze. It was only until these agents were applied topically that the pronounced effect of these agents on the pupil was documented.

Plants of the Solanaceae family that contain these drugs are intricately interwoven with human cultures. This family of plants includes the potato, tomato, chili pepper, and eggplant. It also includes several plants with biological activity in the form of alkaloids contained in leaves, stems, and roots. *Atropa belladonna* contains the alkaloid atropine, an agent that is sometimes used today during cardiopulmonary resuscitation and as premedication prior to anesthesia. Atropa and its closely related plant *Datura stramonium* were used in primitive cultures as hallucinogens and in larger doses as poisons. It is often stated that Julius Caesar poisoned his enemies with *Datura* during his campaign in the northern Alps.

Plants that contain the alkaloids atropine and scopolamine grow as weeds (Jimson weed and Angel's trumpet) throughout the world. Contamination of the fingers with these plants can lead to a transfer of these chemicals onto the corneal surface. The result is a widely dilated pupil that will not contract to bright light. Dilating the pupil with atropine would facilitate cataract surgery or it would also allow patients with central cataracts to have some rudimentary vision by allowing light rays to enter around the periphery of the diseased lens. Although these physicians were unaware of how these plants altered pupil size, it was the exposure of the receptors in the iris that allowed this remarkable effect to take place.

Eventually, curious physicians asked how this plant extract might be producing this action on the pupil, and the answer to that question promoted our understanding of chemical transmission. As early as 1867, J. Bernstein discovered that direct application of atropine to the third nerve did not dilate the pupil and he suggested that the pupillary sphincter must be blocked by interfering with some "mediator substance" between the nerve and the muscle (75). This statement was made over 30 years before the landmark studies by Thomas Elliot and Otto Loewi that led to our understanding of chemical transmission between nerve and muscle and between nerve cells.

The chemical mediator that constricted the pupil by contracting the pupillary sphincter was eventually discovered to be acetylcholine, but several more studies had to explain why this agent would not constrict the pupil when it was applied directly to the cornea. Acetylcholine is rapidly metabolized by cholinesterase, which resides in the corneal epithelium, and so the agent is broken down into inactive metabolites before it can reach the iris. However, the finding that a chemical that resembled acetylcholine was released into the anterior chamber of the eye following stimulation of the ciliary nerve provided strong evidence that the actual chemical transmitter was acetylcholine. Thus, atropine produced mydriasis by blocking the acetylcholine receptors on the iris sphincter.

4.1.3 Pilocarpine

Pilocarpine is an alkaloid isolated from the leaves of *Pilocarpus jaborandi*, native to the Brazilian Amazon basin. The indigenous people used it to induce sweating, and this property encouraged French scientists to find the active ingredient. It also produced extreme miosis. The alkaloid was isolated from the leaves in 1874. Extracts of the leaves were used extensively by John N. Langley when he studied the autonomic nervous system in the late nineteenth century. The plant is harvested from the rain forest, but is not grown commercially. At one time, topical pilocarpine was used to treat glaucoma, but because of side effects, it is rarely used today. The drug produces miosis by stimulating the acetylcholine receptors on the pupillary sphincter.

Pilocarpine eye drops can be used to evaluate the fixed dilated pupil. Dilated pupils are sometimes produced by inadvertent contamination of the conjunctiva by atropine. Dilated pupils are also an ominous sign of brain insults either resulting from a cardiac arrest or from compression of the oculomotor nerve. The use of pilocarpine in deciding between these two etiologies requires placement of dilute pilocarpine onto the surface of the eye. When the dilated pupil results from CNS pathology, dilute pilocarpine will rapidly constrict the pupil. However, if the dilated pupil results from topical application of atropine, there will be no change in the size of the pupil (76). Pilocarpine cannot overcome the blockage of the sphincter by muscarinic antagonists (77). Concentrations of pilocarpine of 0.1 percent are used for this purpose.

4.1.4 Physostigmine

The use of miotics in ophthalmology also has its origins in the plant kingdom. The discovery of physostigmine is historically integrated with the plant *Physostigma venenosum*. In eighteenth-century Nigeria, a red soup made from a bean of this plant was given to suspected witches in a ceremony called "trial by ordeal." The suspected witch would be forced to drink the Calabar bean soup and, if the suspect died, then this proved witchcraft. Survival was equivalent to innocence. British and Portuguese traders who visited Old Calabar, an eastern province of Nigeria in the eighteenth century, observed horrific witch trials, which usually led to a prolonged agonal death, accompanied by convulsions, vomiting, salivation, and respiratory compromise. It is estimated that the "chop nut" (as it was called) accounted for over 100 deaths annually.

In 1858, the Calabar bean was taken to England and studied by Robert Christison in Edinburgh, who ingested the bean and recorded the toxic side effects. In the 1860s, two Scottish ophthalmologists, Thomas Fraser and Douglas Argyll Robertson, described that topical application of the plant extract would constrict the pupil (78). Argyll Robertson proposed that the plant extract, now called physostigmine or eserine, could be used to treat glaucoma by repeated topical applications to keep the pupil in a state of miosis. By that time, it was known that the flow of fluid out of the anterior chamber was enhanced if the pupil was in a constricted state.

The mechanism of action could not be appreciated until the role of acetylcholine in neurochemical transmission had been described. Acetylcholine was subsequently found to be the transmitter released by the parasympathetic nerve endings. Physostigmine is the first of several drugs that have the property of blocking the action of acetylcholinesterase, an enzyme that terminates the action of acetylcholine. Physostigmine was then used to map out the distribution of acetylcholine transmission in the peripheral nervous system. The pupil in this case served as the first demonstration of the cholinergic properties of the drug.

4.1.5 Epinephrine and Phenylephrine

Some of the more interesting chemicals that transmit information in the brain are the amines. An amine is a chemical derivative of ammonia, whereby one of the hydrogen atoms has been replaced by an organic radical. The amines have unique roles to play in behavior and emotion. Some of the more common amines that are discussed in popular science are epinephrine, norepinephrine, dopamine, histamine, and serotonin. These five chemicals are involved in the transmission of information in the central nervous system. Much of what we know about how drugs interact with these chemicals was gained by study of the pupil.

Near the end of the nineteenth century, physiologists were beginning to understand how secretions of fluids in one organ affected other parts of the body, distant from the organ of secretion. Extracts of the adrenal glands were shown to have remarkable effects on the body (including the pupil) by John J. Abel (1857–1938) in 1899. In 1892, Langley and Anderson showed that, in cats, intravenously administered adrenal extracts would dilate the pupil (79). This hormonal influence on the pupil size of cats suggested that adrenal secretion alone could dilate the pupil, although this was not tested in human subjects.

In the cat, epinephrine would dilate the pupil just like stimulation of the sympathetic nerve in the neck. This meant that painful stimuli below a completely transected spinal cord would still have the potential to dilate the pupil if concentrations of certain hormones were elevated via adrenal or other mechanisms. As discussed earlier in this chapter, an astute observation by Elliott led to the early suggestion that a chemical like epinephrine (norepinephrine) was released by the nerve and that it was the agent that acted on the dilator muscle. These experiments with cats led to considerable confusion about the pupillary effects of intravenous sympathomimetics in humans. Investigators later demonstrated that the exquisite sensitivity of the cat iris to circulating catecholamines is not found in primates (80).

In humans, topical application of adrenal extracts or epinephrine onto the surface of the eye was only moderately effective in dilating the pupil. This was paradoxical because other drugs such as atropine, physostigmine, and cocaine would readily produce their pupillary effects by simply applying the agents directly on the cornea. Several years of study were required before it was realized that the cornea provides a barrier to the diffusion of epinephrine, in many ways like that observed for acetylcholine. The actual compound released by sympathetic nerve stimulation is norepinephrine, a drug with a similar chemical structure to epinephrine. Phenylephrine is an alpha 1 adrenergic agonist with a structure like norepinephrine that readily penetrates the cornea and activates the dilator muscle to produce mydriasis.

4.1.6 Nicotine

Tobacco was a traditional American Indian medication that was used during sacred religious ceremonies and to finalize negotiations. It was sent to the court of Catherine de Medici by Jean Nicot in 1559 from Brazil, hence the word nicotine as the active ingredient. Over the years, it became a highly popular recreational drug that has the potential for dependence and tolerance. Nicotine is inhaled from tobacco in the form of cigarettes, cigars, and chewing tobacco. Nicotine is not actually used by physicians today as a drug, except in the form of a nicotine patch to facilitate withdrawal from the use of tobacco. It has several physiological effects in humans, including a heightened awareness, a feeling of contentment, and relaxation.

Measurement of the pupil played a key role in determining nicotine's mechanism of action, but it was not because of topical application of the drug. Langley took up the study of nicotine in 1889 and learned that its effects on the pupil held the key to its mechanism of action. The dilator muscle of the iris is controlled by the sympathetic nerve that originates in the upper thoracic spinal cord. Langley observed that he could block the transmission from the spinal cord to the eye by painting the superior cervical ganglion with nicotine. This produced a Horner's syndrome on that side. He used this information to map out the autonomic nervous system in diverse areas of the body. By painting the ciliary ganglion with nicotine, he demonstrated a widely dilated pupil. This was the first evidence that the ciliary ganglion was a relay station for the pupillary light reflex that traversed the midbrain on its path to the pupillary sphincter. Over the early years of the twentieth century, it was discovered that the autonomic ganglia used the chemical acetylcholine to convey information. These "cholinergic" chemical junctions were then labeled nicotinic junctions because Langley had shown them to be vulnerable to the blocking effect of nicotine (79).

4.1.7 Botulinum Toxin

Botulism is a form of food poisoning caused by a toxin formed by the bacterium *Clostridium botulinum*. The toxin binds to presynaptic cholinergic nerve terminals and decreases the release of acetylcholine. It produces neuromuscular paralysis and interferes with autonomic activity. Botulism blocks both the sympathetic and the parasympathetic innervation of the iris, resulting in mid-position pupils that react poorly to light.

Botox is an injectable form of botulinum toxin that is used to ablate wrinkles around the eye and on the forehead. Periorbital injections of Botox can produce mydriasis by blocking the innervation of the pupillary sphincter. Systemic reactions can occur if Botox is inadvertently injected systemically. Dysphagia and generalized muscle weakness can then be life-threatening.

4.1.8 Brimonidine

Brimonidine is a topical ocular agent that can be used to treat glaucoma. It is an alpha 2 adrenergic agonist with very little affinity for the alpha 1 adrenergic receptor. The drug decreases the production of aqueous humor and lowers intraocular pressure. It will produce constriction of the pupil by preventing the release of norepinephrine from the postsynaptic sympathetic nerves in the iris. It is commonly used in research protocols to produce a pharmacologic "Horner's pupil." Stimulation of a peripheral nerve and the "light off" response in awake subjects will dilate the pupil by contracting the dilator muscle of the iris. Brimonidine partially blocks this response. In patients with Horner's syndrome, the response is blunted, and the test has been suggested as an alternative method to diagnose Horner's syndrome (81).

Apraclonidine is another alpha 2 adrenergic agonist, but compared to brimonidine, it has more potent alpha 1 activity. When this drug is instilled in the affected eye of

Horner's syndrome, it will produce a mild dilation of the pupil because of denervation hypersensitivity of the dilator muscle. When the drug is instilled in a normal eye, there is a small constriction of the pupil, like what is observed after brimonidine. Thus, the topical application of apraclonidine in Horner's syndrome produces a reversal of anisocoria.

4.2 Systemic Drugs and the Size and Reflexes of the Pupil

With the information provided in the previous section, it is possible to predict which systemic drugs will elicit changes in pupil size and reactivity. Both divisions of the autonomic nervous system can be affected by systemic drugs. Although topical application of drugs provides information regarding the chemical transmitters in the iris, the control of pupil size and reactivity involves retinal and central components that are poorly understood. A few of these drugs will be discussed in following paragraphs. Regrettably, there are only a few studies that have utilized infrared pupillometry to study the effect of centrally acting drugs on the pupil. The effects of general anesthesia, opioids, and neuromuscular blocking agents will be discussed in later chapters.

4.2.1 Cholinergic Parasympathetic Agents

Langley demonstrated in 1890 that painting the autonomic ganglia with nicotine would block ganglionic transmission (82–85). Much of this work was performed on the ciliary ganglion and revealed a total loss of the light reflex by application of nicotine. High doses of nicotine will therefore block nicotinic ganglionic transmission. The ciliary ganglia can also be blocked by a class of drugs once used to induce hypotension during anesthesia. During this technique, fixed dilated pupils were observed following administration of hexamethonium, pentolinium, or trimethaphan. These agents block ganglionic nicotinic transmission. This method is rarely used today, but was an alarming sign to practitioners who were unaware of how these drugs affected the pupil. Paradoxically, low systemic doses of nicotine augment transmission in autonomic ganglia. Thus, smoking cigarettes augments transmission in the ciliary ganglion and produces a mild constriction of the pupil (86).

The muscarinic receptor can be blocked or augmented by systemic drugs acting on the pupillary sphincter. Scopolamine and atropine are classic examples that produce mydriasis. Systemic administration does not totally block the light reflex. Agents with mild anticholinergic activity are often used for treatment of Parkinson's disease. Examples are Cogentin (benztropine) and procyclidine; both agents can produce a small pupillary dilation. Other agents with antimuscarinic properties such as dicyclomine and propantheline have not been studied with infrared pupillometry. No study has examined the effect of large doses of antidepressants and antihistamines such as diphenhydramine on pupil size and reactivity. Many antidepressants have antimuscarinic properties and in large doses can produce mydriasis and pupillary areflexia (87).

Agents that enhance cholinergic transmission have been chemically engineered to produce highly toxic poisons. Commonly used insecticides are cholinesterase inhibitors that can be highly toxic to farm workers who are in daily contact with the agents. Agents used in chemical warfare are also often used to contaminate large areas of enemy territory as a means of decimating the population. The poisoning of individuals critical to certain governments has been accomplished by a uniquely developed cholinesterase inhibitor. For example, in August 2020, Alexei Navalny was poisoned with a Novichok nerve agent, a class of poisons derived from cholinesterase inhibitors (The Navalny Case and the German–Russian Relationship at the Limit. *Der Spiegel*, September 24, 2020). These agents are toxic even in small amounts when in contact with the skin. They are lethal through overstimulation of skeletal muscle, interfering with normal ventilation, and death occurs secondary to respiratory failure. Miosis is typically observed prior to cardiovascular collapse.

4.2.2 Adrenergic Sympathetic Agents

Amphetamine is the prototype sympathetic drug that has pupillary activity when given systemically. The drug dilates the pupil and diminishes the magnitude of the pupillary light reflex. The action on the light reflex is thought to be related to increased inhibitory activity in the EW nucleus (39). Methylphenidate has a similar effect on the pupil. Cocaine prevents the uptake of norepinephrine at the alpha 1 adrenergic dilator muscle synapse. The resulting eye sign with dilated pupils and conjunctival hyperemia is sometimes referred to as the "cocaine pupil." Other norepinephrine uptake inhibitors such as amitriptyline can also dilate the pupil in large doses. This class of agents can produce widely dilated pupils with pupillary areflexia, simulating brain death (87).

Adrenergic blockers produce pupillary constriction by blocking dilator muscle function. Typical agents are terazosin, prazosin, and doxazosin. Dexmedetomidine is an unusual drug that constricts the pupil in awake subjects, but increases the magnitude of the light reflex. During anesthesia, it has no effect on pupil size, but increases the light reflex and depresses pupillary reflex dilation (88).

4.2.3 Psychoactive Agents and Hallucinogens

Dopamine antagonists such as droperidol, chlorpromazine, and haloperidol constrict the pupil by an unknown mechanism (89, 90). Attempts to detect unblocked dermatomes during combined epidural–general anesthesia would be difficult if these drugs are given, as discussed in Chapter 9.

The effect of marijuana on the pupil is complex. To date, there is no consensus that indicates a unique effect of marijuana on the pupil or on the pupillary reactions. One study has recently reported an effect on pupillary constriction velocity by delta-9-tetrahydrocannabinol (THC), but this has not been confirmed (91). Others have reported an effect on re-dilation velocity (92). The effect might be related to drug-induced sedation to produce a smaller pupil.

Entrepreneurs have taken up the idea that pupillary reflexes can detect drug effects that predict inability to function optimally in the workplace (e.g., SoberEye Inc.). More importantly, they propose that measurement of the pupil can provide real-time assessment of worker impairment from alcohol, fatigue, and drugs such as marijuana. Such proposals will benefit from more data that will correlate the changes in the pupillary reflexes to motor skills.

The psychedelic drugs act as agonists on serotonin 5HT2A receptors. Examples are LSD, mescaline, psilocybin, and ecstasy. They produce varying degrees of altered consciousness. Although outlawed for public use, except in the state of Oregon where psilocybin is legal, the drugs are still used illegally and in research on depression and mental illness. The prototypical drugs LSD, psilocybin, and ecstasy all produce pupillary dilation, but an analysis of their effect on the light reflex waveform has not been studied (93).

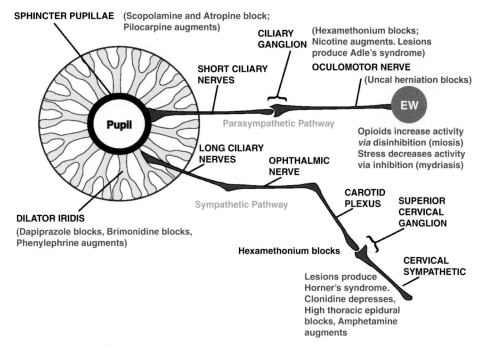

Figure 4.1 This figure illustrates some of the medications that can alter the pupil. Permission for reproduction of image was granted by Wolters Kluwer Health, Inc. License Number: 5592040057072.

LSD increases activity in the locus coeruleus, a nucleus that has been implicated in producing inhibition of the EW nucleus. Figure 4.1 summarizes the locations where drugs and lesions can alter pupil size and pupil reactivity.

Chapter 5

Unusual Pupillary Syndromes

> The pupil of the right eye is very small, and the left pupil is large. The right eyelid is droopy.
>
> (Silas Weir Mitchell, *Gunshot Wounds and Other Injuries of Nerves*, 1864)

The reactions of the pupil have interested countless numbers of medical practitioners and scientists over the past millennium. The history of how this modern view of pupillary behavior evolved can best be appreciated by reading isolated and separate accounts of the various pupillary syndromes that are known to exist. Each syndrome is usually identified by the individual who originally described the clinical signs and symptoms. Pupillary behavior for the physician is only of interest if the patient has somewhat normal pupillary physiology. It is of no use to be testing for the light reflex or reflex dilation of the pupil if the iris is fixed to the lens because of prior eye surgery. For the perioperative intensivist who must occasionally manage critically ill patients, it is important to not be fooled by benign pupillary syndromes that obliterate both the light reflex and reflex dilation. The following syndromes are rare, but should be part of the knowledge base of the clinical pupillometrist. References relating to the origin of these syndromes can be located in the extensive bibliography of Irene Loewenfeld's book (39).

5.1 Argyll Robertson Syndrome

Patients with Argyll Robertson pupils have small pupils that are often distorted and non-reactive to a light stimulus. Before the use of penicillin, a pupil that was nonreactive to light but reacted to near vision was thought to indicate tertiary syphilis. Today, it is recognized that such diverse diseases as diabetes, cerebral hemorrhage, and chronic alcoholism can produce this syndrome. The lesion is located in the pathway from the pretectal nucleus to the EW nucleus. The pupillary near vision fibers are situated more ventrally within the tegmentum and thus escape damage. The presence of an intact near reflex with an absent light reflex is called "light–near dissociation." With attention to the proper settings, it is possible to document the light–near dissociation (Figure 5.1) with both the Neuroptics PLR-3000 and the Algiscan instruments.

Reflex dilation is often lacking in patients with Argyll Robertson pupils. If reflex dilation is used to define sensory levels, it will often be found that the pupils do not dilate to a noxious stimulus, even if opioids have not been given. In addition, the light reflex is absent even before induction of anesthesia and so will not be a rough measure of volatile anesthetic concentrations as it is with other patients. The eye reflexes in patients with this syndrome would not be useful guides in predicting neurologic recovery after traumatic brain injuries or cardiac arrest (see Chapter 11).

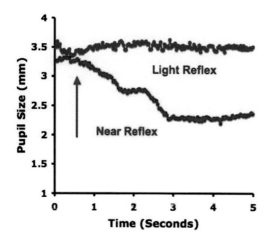

Figure 5.1 Light–near dissociation is characterized by an absent or sluggish light reflex with retention of the near reflex. Tracing from a consenting volunteer subject. Red tracing: Subject changed focus from far to near at time zero. Arrow is approximate latency.

5.2 Spastic Miosis

The pupil in a patient with spastic miosis is small and has diminished light reflexes. In addition, the re-dilation phase of the reflex is sluggish. The only difference between this syndrome and the Argyll Robertson syndrome is the retention of the miotic response to near vision with the latter syndrome. The etiology is the same for both processes, but the lesion is more extensive in spastic miosis and therefore also damages the pathway that contains the near-vision response. As with the Argyll Robertson pupil, reflex dilation may be absent or markedly reduced. Although old age also produces a small pupil, the reactions of the pupil, including the light reflex and reflex dilation, are present in older subjects.

5.3 Glaucoma

In patients with glaucoma, increased pressure within the anterior chamber can dilate the pupil and reduce the extent of the light reflex. The mechanism of these effects is unknown, but may relate to the effect of reduced oxygen supply to the sphincter muscle (94). It is unlikely, however, that the clinician will observe the acute effects of glaucoma because these patients rarely present for elective surgery without a diagnosis, and when the diagnosis is made it is treated by an ophthalmologist. Patients with chronic narrow angle glaucoma, however, are often encountered perioperatively. Modern topical drug treatments for glaucoma include combinations of alpha 2 agonists and beta-blockers such as timolol. However, cholinergic agonists such as pilocarpine and phospholine are still used by some patients. These drugs produce a tightly contracted miotic pupil, and because the iris is limited mechanically, there is usually no observable light reflex. Reflex dilation of the pupil is also absent when these drugs are used to treat glaucoma because the sphincter is unable to relax. Case reports suggest that even brain death does not result in pupillary dilation in patients who have chronically been taking cholinergic agonists for chronic narrow angle glaucoma.

5.4 Adie's Syndrome

The Adie's–Holme's syndrome was described by two neurologists in 1931 (95). It is characterized by a unilateral dilated pupil that constricts sluggishly to light. Typically, the diagnosis is made by a neuro-ophthalmologist who tests for hypersensitivity to dilute concentrations of pilocarpine. The etiology is unknown, but it is thought to result from a lesion in the ciliary ganglion. This lesion explains the absent or reduced light reflex, which must pass through this synaptic relay.

Much confusion exists in the literature as to what pupillary findings are necessary for the diagnosis of Adie's syndrome. The tonic pupil is poorly understood by most clinicians. It is one of the confounding variables in the assessment of pupillary reflexes in a large population of hospitalized patients. The typical patient is a young female with a large nonreactive pupil and absent or reduced deep tendon reflexes. Sluggish contraction to near vision may also be present. The importance for clinicians is to document the presence of Adie's syndrome, so the absent reflex and anisocoria are not cause for alarm during critical illness. The syndrome affects both eyes in 20 percent of cases; because the parasympathetic pathway is damaged, reflex dilation of the pupil will be reduced or absent. The clinical finding of a "light–near" dissociation can also be apparent with Adie's and Parinaud syndromes. Parinaud syndrome is a unique syndrome produced by lesions in the rostral midbrain and is recognized by failure to gaze upward (upgaze paralysis). Thus, to the neuro-ophthalmologist, a "light–near" dissociation has diagnostic implications.

5.5 Chronic Renal Failure and Diabetes

In a typical physician's practice, the disease that most commonly produces abnormal pupillary reflexes is diabetes (96–98). This disease can decrease both the size of the pupil and the extent of the light reflex. There are many factors that contribute to these pupillary changes. The same process that produces the peripheral neuropathy damages the pupillary fibers within the oculomotor nerve. Other factors that decrease the light reflex are damage to the intercalated neuron between the pretectum and the EW nucleus that results in a syndrome very similar to the Argyll Robertson syndrome. The iris stroma becomes rigid because of the vascular changes that occur in prolonged diabetes. Finally, the sympathetic innervation of the radial muscle is defective, and this can be demonstrated by the delay in recovery of pupil diameter following a light flash.

5.6 Horner's Syndrome

This syndrome is familiar to all practicing physicians and is characterized by ptosis, miosis, and unilateral lack of facial sweating. The cause is an interruption of the pathway that innervates the dilator muscle of the iris and is a valuable diagnostic finding because the etiology can have profound implications. In the previous chapter, the role of cocaine in the diagnosis of this syndrome was discussed. A new-onset Horner's syndrome during surgery cannot be appreciated by observation of the pupils because during anesthesia there is no appreciable tone in the dilator muscle of the iris (99).

The behavior of a *chronic* Horner's pupil during surgical anesthesia is unique. Denervation of the dilator muscle induces a postsynaptic receptor that is exquisitely sensitive to circulating catecholamines that have alpha 1 agonist activity. Because the normal innervation of the radial muscle is lacking during general anesthesia, the Horner's pupil becomes somewhat of a bioassay for circulating catecholamines. A case of chronic Horner's syndrome will be presented in Chapter 13 (47).

Rapid increases of desflurane concentration result in elevations of norepinephrine and epinephrine (100). Although there is concomitant pupillary dilation, these hormones do not activate the dilator muslcle. The pupillary dilation is secondary to inhibition of the EW nucleus (99). Thus, without denervation sensitivity, the pupil does not dilate during large increases in adrenergic agonists. However, massive increases of catecholamines during pheochromocytoma resection can, in rare cases, produce unreactive dilated pupils (101).

Horner's syndrome can be caused by an interruption of the sympathetic pathway innervating the iris at three separate locations. A central Horner's syndrome develops when there is interruption in the supraspinal pathway that activates the preganglionic sympathetic neurons in the upper spinal cord. A preganglionic Horner's syndrome is typically caused by a Pancoast tumor in the lung that prevents activation of the sympathetic neurons in the superior cervical ganglion. The postganglionic pathway traverses a circuitous route into the orbit. Hydroxyamphetamine eye drops are used to differentiate preganglionic from postganglionic lesions. This topical drug in a 1 percent concentration will dilate the preganglionic Horner's pupil, but fail to dilate the pupil with postganglionic Horner's. Hydroxyamphetamine releases the norepinephrine that is stored in the presynaptic terminals, but the terminals of postsynaptic lesions do not contain norepinephine and hydroxyamphetamine then fails to dilate the pupil.

5.7 Old Age

Increasing age by itself has little effect on the pupil except for a small decrease in size. Loewenfeld has studied the cause for this relative miosis in the elderly and has concluded that it is most likely caused by decreased tonic inhibition of the EW nucleus (39). This results in a mild decrease in reflex dilation, but this reflex is by no means absent in the elderly. Disease is more prominent in the elderly so that the pupillary abnormalities that occur with chronic alcoholism, diabetes, and post cataract extraction syndromes are therefore more common in this population.

5.8 Aphakia

Absence of the intraocular lens is a consequence of surgical treatment for cataract. Before the widespread use of lens phacoemulsification, the surgical technique for cataract extraction involved incising the iris (iridectomy), grasping, then extracting, the lens with a special scapula. Older patients today that have had this surgical procedure can have immobile pupils secondary to the iridectomy or to adhesions that form between the iris and the implanted lens. Modern cataract surgery avoids interference with pupillary mobility. The technique involves a small incision in the cornea, emulsification of the lens within the capsule, then extraction of the lens material and implantation of the new lens within the lens capsule. The new lens can often be seen with the unaided eye during examination of the pupils, and, if observed closely, it will be appreciated that no iridectomies or lack of pupillary reflexes are apparent.

5.9 Relative Afferent Pupillary Defect

The term "relative afferent pupillary defect" or RAPD refers to a defect in the transmission of the afferent light stimulus on one side as compared to the other. The lesion is usually in the optic nerve, but can be at any location between the light signal and the pretectal nucleus. For example, an opaque cornea or lens on one side can produce RAPD, as can unilateral optic neuritis or retinal disease. Head trauma can produce RAPD by damage to the orbit or optic nerve.

The clinical diagnosis of RAPD is made with the "swinging light test" first described by P. Levatin in 1959 (102). As one moves a bright light from one eye to the other, it will be noticed that the side with RAPD will dilate instead of constrict as the light is moved onto that eye. This occurs because the light stimulus is producing less pupillomotor effect on that side.

The practical value of this reflex for the intensivist is during the examination of head-injured patients who are either sedated or comatose. Visual acuity is commonly used to assess traumatic injuries to the globe that might result in retinal hemorrhage or optic nerve injury, but this may be difficult to assess in the obtunded patient. The swinging light test can be quantitated in these patients, and a significant RAPD suggests damage to some portion of the afferent limb of the light reflex on the affected eye. Damage to the occipital lobe will affect vision, but should not produce an afferent defect.

The swinging light test is a valuable tool because it tests the relative integrity of the afferent arc of the pupillary light reflex. Simply comparing the quality of the light reflex between the two eyes does not accomplish that purpose. A diminished reflex on one side compared to the other eye can be because either the afferent signal is blocked or the efferent third nerve is blocked.

The dilation of the pupil that occurs in the eye with the defective afferent light signal is dependent on an active inhibitory process at the EW nucleus at the time of the test. This implies that the test would be difficult to perform in patients who have been treated with opioids in sufficient doses to produce pupillary constriction. The same issue would arise during general anesthetics that produce miosis.

5.10 Autoimmune and Neurodegenerative Disorders

Certain rare autoimmune and neurodegenerative disorders can result in loss of skeletal motor function, sometimes associated with depressed pupillary reactivity. Amyotrophic lateral sclerosis and the syndromes of Guillain–Barré and Miller Fisher are examples (103–105). Nonreactive pupils have been reported with these diseases. The lesion in Miller Fisher syndrome is in the ciliary ganglion or at the neuromuscular junction of the iris sphincter. The electroencephalogram can confirm the diagnosis of cognitive–motor dissociation when there is complete muscular paralysis. Pupillary examinations in many of these reports were conducted using a pen light. There are no reports of using portable infrared pupillometry on these cases when the light reflex was reported to be absent with the pen light. It is possible that with this new technology, small residual reflexes would be observed.

Measurement of the Pupil

In all the accumulating volumes of loose medical literature, no symptom has been more loosely treated as the size of the pupil. Off-hand decisions in this matter, such as commonly made, and their usual records "pupils dilated" or "pupils constricted," are at best useless, and often deceiving.

(Edward Jackson, MD, Determination of the Size of the Pupil. *Proceedings of the Philadelphia County Medical Society*, 8:105–108, 1888)

6.1 Commercial Pupillometers

The pupil can be seen but not touched or connected directly to recording devices. Casual observation of the pupil therefore comes to us only through our own vision, through our own pupils. But this presents a difficult challenge. The pupillary reactions are too fast to be quantitated by a mm rule or a dot comparison device. Shining light in the pupil to visualize it alters not only the resting size of the pupil, but also the sensitivity of the retina. This makes measurements of the pupil a nearly impossible portion of human anatomy to study. The pupil is nothing, a void. No wonder that precise methods to study the physiology and pharmacology of the pupil began to emerge only in the twentieth century.

When discussing pupillometers, the question often arises as to what is meant by the word "portable." Bulky and expensive desktop infrared pupillometers are available for use by neuro-ophthalmologists. They cannot be brought to the bedside or into the operating room or emergency room. Smaller units have a lightweight goggle-type eyepiece that is attached to a laptop computer. The "Eye Check" is one such instrument that is used to "detect drug impairment." This instrument requires full patient cooperation and could not be used in uncooperative subjects or those heavily sedated or under general anesthesia. Adaptica Srl (Padua, Italy) produces an instrument that can measure the light reflex, but it requires an awake subject. These instruments might be considered portable because they are small enough to be transported around the hospital. However, they do require some set-up time and are therefore not acceptable for routine use. On the other extreme are instruments that use comparison discs, rulers, or black dots. These devices are used either with an attached light or with a separate pen light, but do not provide true objective measurements (15, 47, 106).

For clinical use, certain requirements should be satisfied. The device should have a recharging module conveniently located to serve both as a recharging station and as a dedicated location for all providers who might use the instrument. Battery life should be long enough to last for at least two hours. It should provide an objective readout that is retained in the memory of the same device with each measurement time stamped and

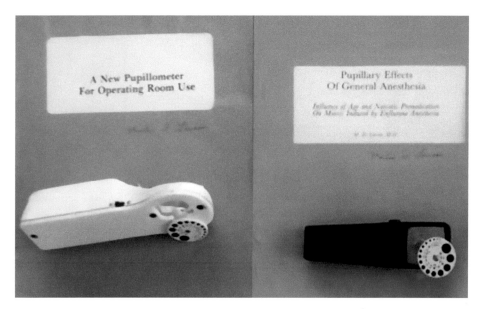

Figure 6.1 Dot-comparison pupillometers constructed by the author to measure changes in pupil size and reactivity during anesthesia (114). Photograph by author.

dated. Any portion of the portable instrument that touches the patient should initially be sterile and thereafter only used for that same patient. The instrument should be small enough to be easily carried by hand or in a lab-coat pocket.

Several dot-comparison pupillometers have been described (Figure 6.1), with the first for use in anesthesia described by Dudley W. Buxton (1855–1931) in 1888. None of these instruments would allow an objective measure of the light reflex. Ambient light cannot be controlled unless there is accurate control of the room lights. For pupil size measurements, dot-comparison pupillometers are only marginally superior to unaided visual assessments.

A slight advancement is made by instruments such as the Elsinor pupillometer (107) that superimposes the image of the pupil on a mm scale. This instrument blocks out the ambient light and is thereby useful for size determinations in the absence of the confounding variable of room light. Without a means of recording phasic pupillary activity, they cannot be used to assess either the light reflex or reflex pupillary dilation. Infrared pupillometry to assess the dynamic properties of the light reflex dates back nearly 100 years. Visible photography had the limitation of light-induced changes in the size of the pupil. Infrared light does not alter pupil size and was used by Otto Lowenstein as early as 1926 (Figure 6.2) to begin the modern era of pupillometry (39).

Objective measurement of the pupil that benefits the clinician as described in this book requires some form of electronic instrumentation. Many different pupillometers are available and more are devised each year. One must first ask what pupillary parameters are of interest and what degree of accuracy is required. Clearly, an instrument that measures only static pupillary diameter would have limited use if either the light reflex or reflex dilation were of interest. Also, an instrument that can detect only 0.5–1 mm changes is of limited use. Control of ambient light is essential with any pupillometric technique.

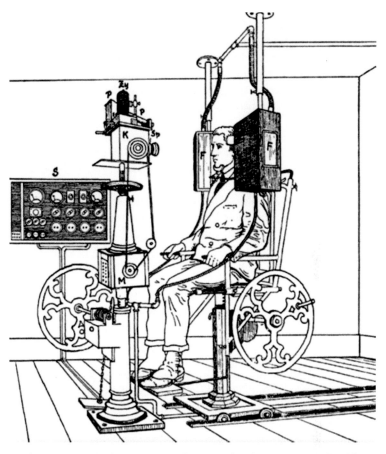

Figure 6.2 With the Lowenstein photographic pupillometer, infrared images were analyzed for pupil size by visually inspecting each individual photographic image. Permission for reproduction of image obtained from Wolters Kluwer Health, Inc. License Number: 5614231355848.

With the pupillometer illustrated in Figure 6.1, the pupil size could be measured to within 0.2 mm. This device allowed some preliminary investigations on the pupillary size changes that occurred during the induction of anesthesia with thiopental. Thiopental produced a small initial dilation that was also blocked by meperidine premedication (see next chapter). The pupil constricted to the same small diameter of around 2 mm whether meperidine was given or not given prior to thiopental (15). This was unique information, but it had little practical value and it provided no opportunity to examine the dynamic features of the reflexes. Furthermore, there was no permanent record that could be analyzed.

6.2 Portable Infrared Pupillometers

The first Fairville portable infrared pupillometer was constructed by Elliot Carter in 1983. This pupillometer used a laptop computer connected with a long cable to a hand-held optical device that was positioned over the eye. The light stimulus was provided by an array of green-light-emitting diodes that surrounded the image processor. The initial manuscript on the use of this instrument is from 1989 (108). This small case series demonstrated the typical changes that occurred during a routine halothane anesthetic. Only 20 cases were described, but it was the beginning of an objective measure of the pupil in anesthetized humans. The study demonstrated that thiopental produced a reduction in the extent of the light reflex, that succinylcholine did not block the reflex, that surgical stimulation dilated the pupil, and that fentanyl blocked the dilation. Also with the same instrument, Wallace Pickford studied the light reflex changes brought about by buprenorphine (109).

Several iterations of the original instrument were made to improve image quality and ease of use. Although the Fairville instrument was used in several studies, it was never truly portable because it required a laptop computer to function properly. For example, it was not possible to use it in the hospital except in locations where the small laptop computer could be carried and placed next to the patient. It worked well in the operating room when the laptop computer could be safely placed on the anesthesia machine. Keeler Optical instruments used the Fairville technology to make a truly portable instrument, but it was not accurate enough for clinical use. Current portable pupillometers are highly accurate. Precision of the new devices has been tested by calibrating their pupil diameter readings to known fixed diameter apertures.

Portable pupillometers that measure the light reflex include not only the infrared devices such as Neuroptics and Neurolight, but also the smart-phone-based pupill-ometers (Figure 6.3) that use visible light, such as the Bright Lamp, SoberEye, SmartPupil, Bencom, and Sensitometer devices. These smart phone devices would be more useful if they used infrared light to measure the pupil (110). Also, an algorithm should be embedded in the phone to quantitate the strength of the light reflex (see below). These smart phone pupillometers might soon be perfected to provide useful information, but interpretation of the measurements would still be required by the clinician (111, 112).

Each new smart phone device should have its reliability tested by independent investigators. One smart phone pupillometer has not been able to replicate consistent

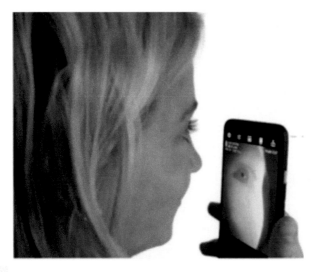

Figure 6.3 Several iterations of smart phone pupillometers have been described. The clinical application of these devices will require independent comparisons to commercially available portable infrared pupillometers. Consent from the author of references 111 and 112.

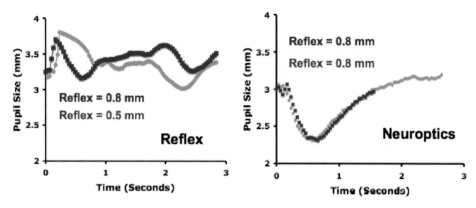

Figure 6.4 Two different pupillometers took sequential measurements on the same patient with identical light sources. The device that was used on the left was a smart phone instrument (Brightlamp), whereas the device used on the right was a portable infrared pupillometer (Neuroptics). Clearly, the smart phone device was unable to repeat accurate measurements. Permission to reproduce image was granted from Future Medicine and the *Journal of Concussion* Attribution 4.0 International CC BY 4.0.

reflexes on the same subject and does not compare to the accuracy of the infrared pupillometers (Figure 6.4; 113).

As currently manufactured, portable infrared pupillometers flood the iris with infrared light, and then measure the reflected image on a microprocessor. The pupil is a hole within this image and can be readily measured as either area or diameter. Measurements can be taken in total darkness if the opposite eye is covered. Portable instruments are available for either the unconscious or conscious subject. Safe infrared radiation levels are determined by the American Conference of Governmental Industrial Hygienists (ACGIH) and the current available instruments are well below the recommended safe levels for continuous exposure. Complications from intermittent measurements have not been reported. Of course, leaving the eye open after a measurement during anesthesia would be hazardous.

The technology of portable infrared pupillometers has been advancing rapidly, and the instruments that are available today will be significantly improved over the next five years. AMTech (Weinheim, Germany) makes pupillometers that scan at 250 Hz and are accurate to 0.1 mm. This instrument would be ideal for use in the hospital, except for the fact that it can be cumbersome to use there because it must be connected to a laptop computer. Obviously, in the unconscious subject, any heavy object that might inadvertently fall on the exposed eye might produce significant injury. Because of this risk, the author has not used this instrument, although it is reported to perform very well in the awake subject.

Because portable instruments attempt to describe very subtle reactions of the pupil, it is essential that hand motions of the examiner and eye movements of the subject will not confound the true pupillary diameter changes. The Neuroptics portable instrument was introduced in 1995 and incorporates pupillary tracking software so that each measurement always fixates on the actual aperture during the time of the measurement. The result is that these instruments provide very precise readings during movement. This can be readily confirmed by comparing the instrumental reading with metal holes of known

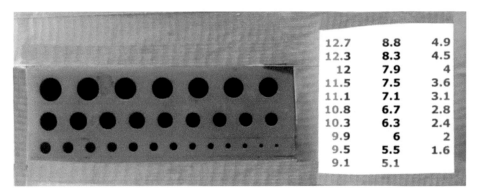

12.7	8.8	4.9
12.3	8.3	4.5
12	7.9	4
11.5	7.5	3.6
11.1	7.1	3.1
10.8	6.7	2.8
10.3	6.3	2.4
9.9	6	2
9.5	5.5	1.6
9.1	5.1	

Figure 6.5 This calibrated tool ensures the stability and accuracy of pupillometer measurements. It calculates the degree of noise with different instruments. The tool is an ordinary holder of metal drill bits. Light reflexes should measure zero and pupillary unrest values should be 0.04 AU or below; see later discussion of PUAL indicating that there is a minimal amount of noise in the pupillometer. Photograph by author.

diameter that are slowly moved during the measurement (Figure 6.5). In addition, portable instruments described in this book have optical corrections that compensate for the variability in vertex distance between subjects.

Neuroptics has several portable pupillometers on the market. One model (VIP-300) is designed to measure pupil size, and the more popular model (NPi-300) is used for measurement of pupil size and the pupillary light reflex. The Neuroptics NPi-300 model uses a cheek rest that stores several measurements that can be downloaded onto the hospital record. This pupillometer is basically a point-and-shoot device that is easy to use and gives a rapid assessment of the quality of the light reflex. Neuroptics has developed an algorithm that purportedly provides an indication of the quality of the light reflex. Prior to infrared techniques, it was common to use the terms such as sluggish, brisk, or absent. The Neurological Pupillary index (NPi) is a proprietary number developed by Neuroptics that is intended to replace these terms with more objective data. The NPi is scaled from 0 to 5, with 0 designating an absent reflex. More extensive discussions of the NPi number will be presented in Chapters 7 and 8. The NPi should not be confused with the National Provider Identification number (NPI). The NPI is a unique number assigned to all healthcare providers.

The Neuroptics PLR-3000 device is ideal for retrieving the many parameters (see Chapter 8) that can be derived from infrared pupillometric techniques (Figure 6.6). The instrument can be programmed to deliver long duration light stimuli and provide continuous measurements in darkness and/or dim to bright light. There are five options to set the timing and illumination for each measurement (see Glossary for discussion of illumination). The parameters of the light reflex are shown on the screen after each measurement. An important feature is the ability to trend several measurements from the same subject.

The ID Med medical device company located in Marseilles, France, makes portable pupillometers (Figure 6.7). The Neurolight instrument measures the light reflex, pupillary unrest (PUAL), and pupillary reflex dilation. A more advanced instrument measures those three parameters plus a value called the Pupillary Pain Index (PPI). The idea of the PPI is to stimulate with tetanic currents through surface electrodes with increasing current intensities. The current begins at the low current value of 10 milliamps and

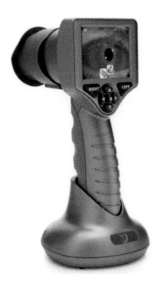

Figure 6.6 The Neuroptics PLR-3000 pupillometer can be programmed to adjust flash intensity, duration of measurement, and background light. The rubber eyecup can be sterilized. Permission from Neuroptics to reproduce image.

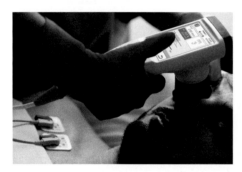

Figure 6.7 The AlgiScan pupillometer includes a Tetanus feature that stimulates selected dermatomes during the pupillary measurement. Permission from ID Med to reproduce image.

then increases in 10-milliampere steps until the pupil dilates 13 percent above baseline. It is a novel concept that is purported to assess the nociception–antinociception balance and/or a measure of opioid effect. The use of the PPI will be discussed in the section on Pupillary Reflex Dilation.

The ID Med instrument called the Algiscan has another feature called "Tetanus." The Tetanus mode of operation provides a 5-second stimulus of a predetermined current setting. This is a useful iteration that allows the testing of blocked and unblocked dermatomes during combined regional–general anesthesia. The PPI and Tetanus features are incorporated into the AlgiScan pupillometer, but are only sold in the United States to investigators who have approved research protocols. The Neurolight does not have the Tetanus feature and is approved for distribution in the United States.

Pupil Size

Dirkovitch saw the marks, and the pupils of his eyes dilated – also his eyes dilated and his face changed.

(Rudyard Kipling, *The Man Who Was*)

7.1 Pupil Size in the Awake State

In the awake condition, there are several indications for measuring the size of the pupil. One common example is to determine pupil size prior to refractive surgery or during the fitting of contact lenses. The portable infrared pupillometers are ideal for this purpose because light can be controlled, and these devices provide consistent reliable measurements (115). The VIP-300 Neuroptics device can be used in total darkness or with an adjustable background illumination. Pupil size is also important as a parameter to trend over time because it can detect a progression of intracranial pathology and/or drug effect. Pupil size is equal in both eyes, although a variable size difference of 0.4 mm diameter is considered within the range of normal. Size difference above 0.4 mm is called anisocoria, discussed in Chapter 13.

Pupil size can be measured in mm diameter or in mm^2 as area. The most common measure reported in the literature is the diameter. To follow a trend of pupil sizes over time, it is advisable to use the same technique for each measurement. Pupil size for *research* purposes is usually measured in the dark-adapted eye with the subject focusing on a distant dim point source of light. This method removes the two variables, ambient light and near fixation, both of which can constrict the pupil. Dark measurements in the office or hospital can be retrieved by turning off room lights and blocking outside light. Alternatively, the opposite eye can be covered, and an occlusive cup placed over the measured eye. But dark adaption takes a variable amount of time that is unique to the patient and the ambient light in the room. Many patients are uncomfortable with pupillary examinations that exceed 10 seconds. That length of time is not sufficient for complete dark adaption. At 15 seconds, dark adaption is over 90 percent complete, but this depends on the amount of photopigment bleach prior to the measurement (39). Because of the importance of trending pupil size, it is important to document accurate and consistent measurements.

Different levels of measurement complexity can provide progressively more information to the clinician. The most convenient measure of pupil size is to use either the NPi device (Neuroptics) or the Neurolight device (ID Med). Measuring the light reflex and pupil size with these point-and-shoot instruments is convenient and rapid.

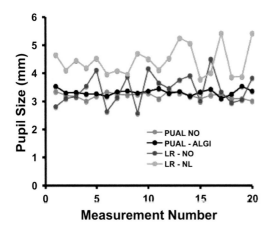

Figure 7.1 The Neuroptics PLR-3000 (NO) and the AlgiScan (Algi) in PUAL mode were used to take 10-second measurements with one eye covered and the measured eye illuminated with approximately 400 lux. As can be observed, repeated measurements were stable over 20 measurements taken over approximately 1 hour. The measurements were taken in ambient room light ranging from 150 to 500 lux. The NPi and Neurolight pupillometer diameter readings were not as consistent. The sequential pupil size measurements taken with the PUAL labels were consistent with repeat measurements. The sequential pupil size measurements taken with the NPi device LR – (NO) and the Neurolight LR – (NL) demonstrated wide scatter when repeat measurements were taken. Measurements taken from consenting volunteer.

More accurate and consistent measurements of pupil size can be accomplished by using the Neuroptics PLR-3000. A low-level background light from the pupillometer can be directed into one eye with the other eye covered. This provides a reference to be compared to previous or future measurements without concern about variable light levels. With this described technique, repeated measures of pupil size are consistently the same even when the measurements are taken in different locations with variable room light. In contrast, the NPi-300 cannot reproduce highly consistent readings at different locations because the measured eye is not totally occluded. The Neurolight device occludes both eyes, but the speed of dark adaption can confound repeated readings (Figure 7.1).

A more advanced method would detect the "light off" (LO) and pupillary unrest in ambient light (PUAL) parameters discussed in Chapter 10. This type of program would document the pupil size, PUAL, and the light off response in a 10-second measurement. Using this method would reveal whether the pupil is fixed either from the various syndromes discussed in Chapter 5 or from opioid medication. The Neuroptics PLR-3000 program in this case would be a 10-second scan with light off at 5 seconds and a background set at 50 microwatts (see Figure 10.17).

When measured with any of these described methods, the size of the pupil can be of value. Drug therapies and traumatic brain injuries, for example, can produce gradual changes in pupil size. A scopolamine patch is another example. Migration of the drug, systemic absorption, or hand contamination from the patch onto the iris sphincter can dilate the pupil by blocking the muscarinic receptor. This produces a slow dilation of the pupil that is unilateral if the drug is locally spread, but bilateral if it results from systemic absorption.

7.2 Pupil Size During Sleep and Anesthesia

The size of the pupil in the awake state is controlled by the influence of light, near fixation, pain, emotions, drugs, muscular activity, perception of brightness, and mental tasks. Because of the many factors that control pupil size, it becomes difficult to ascertain at any one moment which dominant factor is controlling the size of the pupil. The clinician is advised to use the same method for sequential measurements and thereby eliminate many of the confounding factors. The influences that affect pupil size can be minimized during general anesthesia using infrared pupillometry. Subjects are not awake, so pain, near fixation, and muscular activity can be controlled. Light can be excluded. It is therefore of interest how pupil size changes as subjects pass into slow-wave sleep, or during the induction of general anesthesia.

Portable instruments are commonly used in settings that involve patients who are asleep secondary to sedative drug therapy. This is a topic that is rarely discussed in the general medical literature. One of the first anesthetic agents was diethyl ether, which was an unusual agent because it dilated the pupil during deep levels of anesthesia. The agent is no longer in use, but this progressive dilation was undoubtedly related to mobilization of various stress hormones in the central nervous system such as dopamine and norepinephrine as the anesthetic deepened. Ether stress is an experimental entity that has been used to delineate the hormonal responses to stressful stimuli (116).

Modern anesthetic agents such as the barbiturates propofol and sevoflurane do not typically dilate the pupil. After a brief dilation that corresponds to the excitement phase of anesthetic induction, the pupils constrict, and this constriction occurs even in total darkness (15). This unusual behavior of the pupil during anesthetics requires some explanation because it is unlike the reaction of the pupil in the awake state, when the pupils dilate up to 6 or 7 mm in total darkness. The explanation for this difference is the presence of inhibitory influences on the EW nucleus during wakefulness. These inhibitory inputs diminish the firing rate of the EW neurons and in darkness the pupil dilates. But during anesthesia this inhibition is lacking and in the absence of light the EW neurons revert to their spontaneous firing rate. Pupillary constriction or the miosis of sleep is the result. A similar observation was made nearly 300 years ago by Fontana, who observed that during sleep, the pupils of cats became miotic even in darkness. Furthermore, the pupils dilated widely during awakening and the light reflex was then briefly inhibited (31). The pupillary aperture is also constricted during slow-wave sleep in humans (39).

It is known that the onset of natural sleep miosis coincides with eye closure and loss of consciousness. This pupillary constriction is brought about by a combination of loss of sympathetic tone and removal of inhibition at the EW nucleus. So miosis occurs at the onset of sleep (Figure 7.2; 117).

The timing of miosis related to loss of consciousness during anesthesia is not the same as that occurring during natural sleep. As illustrated in Figure 7.3, the pupil contracts to sizes between 2 and 2.5 mm after intravenous induction, but there is a delay of several minutes before this basal diameter is attained (15). Why there is this delay in pupillary constriction with the induction of anesthesia has not been explained. It is generally accepted that a brief period of excitement precedes the development of surgical levels of anesthesia, possibly through a mechanism of disinhibition.

The small pupil after induction of anesthesia and before surgical stimulation is observed in light or dark. There is no appreciable "light off" reflex, but the light reflex is present. Consideration of this process by several investigators has led to the conclusion that the miosis of modern anesthesia develops because of the loss of inhibition combined with intrinsic pacemaker activity within the EW nucleus (see further in Chapter 10; 39).

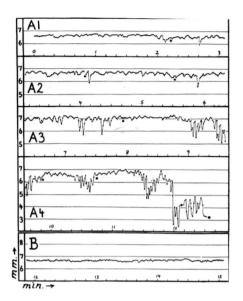

Figure 7.2 This recording is taken from a sleepy human subject prior to and at the time of loss of consciousness at the 12th minute in the A4 segment. Note that as the subject loses consciousness, there is a rapid onset of miosis that is not observed during intravenous inductions. Consent was obtained for reproduction of this image from the Association for Vision and Ophthalmology. License Number: 1422529-1.

7.3 Conditions That Affect the Size of the Pupil

An important issue with any measure derived from the pupil is that an isolated measure has little value compared to repeated measures over time. A one-time measure documents the characteristics of that patient's baseline value. As the patient then progresses into the treatment regimen, the trending of pupillary measurements can be compared to the initial measurements. Importantly, the pupil does not diagnose any disease. It is simply another measurement that the clinician can evaluate along with the other laboratory tests and physical findings that can be observed from that patient.

It is noted that there have been publications that have implicated the value of pupil size in the estimation of intelligence (118), sexual preference, and the risk of cardiac disease. These studies require strict control of lighting conditions and careful averaging methods. More recently, pupil size has been promoted to predict unfavorable outcome in Covid-19 patients (119). These applications of pupil size measurements will require confirmatory studies. Other important scenarios that call for a measure of pupil size are traumatic brain injury, opioid use, postischemic brain stem insults, poisoning following the use of anticholinesterase inhibitors, and intraoperative efficacy of regional analgesia during combined techniques. These issues will be discussed more completely in subsequent chapters.

Although it is commonly thought that hypoxia dilates the pupil, this has never been demonstrated experimentally in human subjects. Volunteers breathing hypoxic mixtures exhibit no change in pupil size or the pupillary light reflex (120). In this study published as an abstract, arterial samples from the volunteers were used to measure oxyhemoglobin saturations (Figure 7.4).

It is clear, however, that more extreme degrees of hypoxia or the addition of hypercapnia (asphyxia) produces pupillary dilation. The neurons in the EW nucleus require oxygen and glucose to function and their activity falls to zero when those conditions are not met. Pupillary dilation and areflexia were commonly observed during

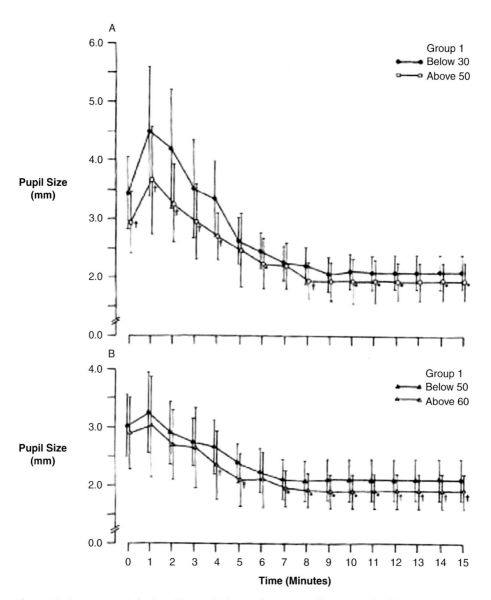

Figure 7.3 A: Intravenous induction without opioid premedication typically results in a brief dilation with a slow pupillary constriction to between 2 and 2.5 mm. Pupil sizes are smaller in the older population. B: With opioid premedication, the initial dilation is absent, but the eventual size is roughly the same. This constriction of the pupil does not apply to induction of anesthesia with ketamine. In both A and B, the data points and the line for patients younger than age 50 are above the data points for patients older than 50. The author's figure is copied from the cited article in *Anesthesiology Review*. McNamara Publishing Company, Inc.

induction of anesthesia with 100 percent nitrous oxide associated with anoxia and hypoventilation (121, 122).

In the older literature on cardiac resuscitation, it was common to advise frequent assessments of pupil size as a measure of cardiac output. Animal studies confirm that the

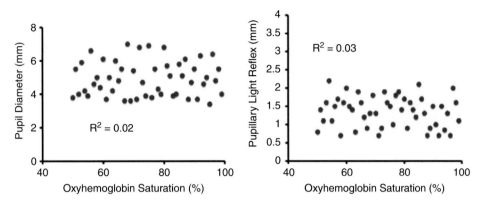

Figure 7.4 Hypoxia produced by breathing hypoxic mixtures to oxyhemoglobin saturations as low as 50 percent have no effect on pupil size or the pupillary light reflex. Modification of figure from cited abstract.

pupil dilates as coronary perfusion pressure falls to low levels (123). In actual clinical practice, this is only partially true because there have been reports of failed resuscitation and brain death in patients with miotic pupils (124). These cases can be observed in patients taking topical agents that produce miosis as a treatment for glaucoma.

There is a surge of epinephrine when cardiac output falls to zero, which often results in pupillary dilation (125). After several minutes, the pupils then constrict into midposition, between 3 and 5 mm in diameter. Pupil size measurements during ACLS as a measure of neurologic outcome are not as valuable as measurements of the pupillary light reflex (124). The light reflex as a measure of clinical outcomes during and after cardiac arrest will be discussed in Chapter 11.

8

Pupillary Light Reflex

In front of the vitreous there is a thin structure that is smooth anteriorly. The color is not the same in all bodies; sometimes it is very black and sometimes less so. In the middle, facing the glassy humor, it has a hole which sometimes dilates, sometimes constricts, as the glassy humor (lens) needs light; it constricts when the light is bright and dilates in darkness. The hole is called the pupil.

(Abu Bakr Muhammad ibn Zakariya al-Razi (Rhazes), *In Liber ad Almansorem*)

8.1 Introduction to the Light Reflex

The pupillary light reflex is often considered the most important reflex in the human body. Measuring the quality of this reflex is the primary reason that portable pupillometers are used. When present, pupillary light reflex signifies life, and when absent it can signify intracranial pathology, cardiac arrest, total spinal, severe drug intoxication, or brain death. There is a diagnostic aphorism stating that coma with an intact pupillary light reflex suggests either metabolic or drug-induced coma, whereas coma associated with an absent pupillary light reflex suggests a structural intracranial lesion (12).

It is important to note that the tonic pupil (see Chapter 5) will not react briskly to the brief light stimulus provided by the portable pupillometers. When an absent reflex is observed with the pupillometer, it is advisable to test the reflex with a long duration light exposure with a pen light to ascertain if a slowly developing constriction of the pupil can be observed (126). Alternatively, the Neuroptics PLR-3000 device can be set for a long duration 180-microwatt light stimulus. A 15-second measurement with the light on would show a gradual slow constriction of the tonic pupil that would not be apparent with a shorter stimulus. Repeat measurements are advised if the pupillometer designates an absent reflex, and visual inspection of the waveform is essential.

Observation of an absent light reflex has significant clinical implications. It is a necessary (but not sufficient) condition for the diagnosis of brain death. Even a weak light reflex signifies an alive patient. In ambiguous cases, an intact light reflex might prevent the need for more costly and time-consuming procedures such as angiography, evoked potentials, and apnea testing (see introduction to Chapter 14).

The Neuroptics NPi instruments stimulate with light for 800 msec and measure for 3 seconds, whereas the Neurolight stimulates for 1 second and measures for 4 seconds. Illumination at the corneal surface is similar with both instruments at approximately 1,000 lux. These pupillometers also present a parameter that is meant to indicate the

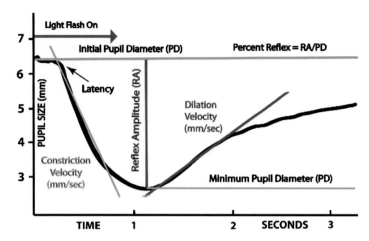

Figure 8.1 As demonstrated in this figure, several parameters can be measured from the light reflex waveform when using portable instruments. Reproduced with the consent of Elsevier under the terms of the Creative Commons CC BY License.

quality of the reflex. The two instruments retrieve similar values when sequential measurements are taken. With these settings, several indices can be retrieved from the light reflex waveform. Absolute constriction amplitude in mm, percent constriction, constriction velocity, dilation velocity, and latency are commonly measured (Figure 8.1).

The clinical implications of the separate values from the waveform are under study by several investigators. Depressed percent reflex and depressed dilation velocity as measured in the PACU have been reported to predict postoperative delirium (127). The early portion of the light reflex is predominately generated by excitation of the EW nucleus, whereas the re-dilation phase is a complicated process that involves inhibition of the EW nucleus and tension in the dilator muscle (128). Several investigators have noted the prognostic value of dilation velocity for the prediction of delirium (129, 130). Depressed light reflexes during cardiac surgery are associated with postoperative delirium (131). Studies that focus on one aspect of the waveform to predict perioperative complications will require confirmation from other research centers.

8.2 The Effect of Pupil Size

The quality of the pupillary light reflex is a topic that requires an extensive discussion. Of all the measures derived from portable pupillometers, the strength of the light reflex has received the most attention in the literature. The archaic descriptions of brisk, sluggish, or absent light reflexes are too subjective as a measure to trend over time. An important confounder in many previous studies was how to evaluate the strength of the light reflex when there is a change in the size of the pupil. Clearly, when the pupil changes size, there are changes in the mechanical features of the iris structure. For example, the 6-mm pupil can easily constrict 2 mm in amplitude, an extent that would be impossible for any pupil sizes below 2 mm. So, if the pupil changes size, then the light reflex changes might occur solely because of iris mechanics. In addition, the amount of light that falls on the retina depends on pupil size. Irene Loewenfeld examined these issues in classic papers from

1971 (132, 133). The interpretation of many older articles on the light reflex is therefore confounded by the question of how much of the depressant change in light reflex extent (amplitude) was due to the change in pupil size. Consequently, the magnitude of the pupillary light reflex has little meaning by itself.

To deal with this problem, the Neuroptics NPi-300 pupillometer has an embedded algorithm that purports to evaluate the quality of the light reflex that is independent from pupil size. The NPi is a dimensionless value from 0 to 5 with any values below 3 considered to be abnormal and 0 to be an absent reflex. This is a proprietary algorithm to Neuroptics that has not been published, but is calculated from the various parameters of the light reflex waveform, including pupil size and constriction velocity. The ID Med pupillometer called the Neurolight presents a similar 1–5 scale that is used to signify the quality of the light reflex. This scale has been termed the QPi or quality of the reflex. This is a new concept for the Neurolight and this author is not aware of any testing in a comparison with the NPi.

Even though the NPi concept is a real innovation, it can provide erroneous values in some unique circumstances. A rapid change in light intensity will produce alterations in pupil size and in the sensitivity of the photoreceptors. Pupil size changes are rapid and begin within less than a second after a change in light directed into the pupil. On the other hand, the sensitivity of the photoreceptors is slower to develop. The discrepancy between the size of the pupil and the response of the photoreceptors can alter the relationship between pupil size and percent reflex so that the NPi is temporarily altered. For example, when the NPi is measured in bright light, the pupil is small, and the reflex is small because of the limitation on iris movement. When the light is then turned off and the subject eye is then in typical relative darkness, the pupil will dilate rapidly, but the photoreceptors are still adapted to the light. Consequently, the pupillary light reflex will be of a smaller amplitude for that pupil size and the NPi will accordingly decrease. The effect, however, is temporary and, within a few minutes, the NPi will gain in value to attain the same value as was observed in bright light (Figure 8.2). It is also important to stress that the NPi values of the tonic pupil as discussed in Chapter 5 will be depressed. These depressed reflexes will be present regardless of traumatic brain injury or drug therapy.

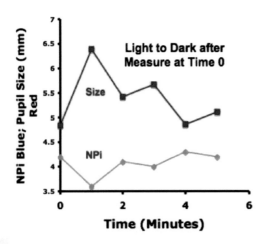

Figure 8.2 A rapid change from light to dark can transiently depress the NPi. The pupil dilates at a more rapid pace than adaption of the photoreceptors. Graph constructed from measurements taken from a consenting volunteer.

More research will be required to reach a consensus on this complex topic. It is possible that the NPi parameter is not the final statement on this issue. Future studies will hopefully clarify the most appropriate algorithm to measure the quality of the pupillary light reflex. The following discussion will present one approach to think about this topic.

8.3 The Importance of Percent Reflex

A portable pupillometer should ideally provide a measure of the light reflex that is independent of the pupil size. Percent reflex is calculated as the constriction amplitude in mm divided by pupil size. This parameter has been used to overcome the effect that pupil size has on the quality of the light reflex. A curve relating pupil size to percent reflex can be constructed by shining a light of variable intensity in one eye and measuring the light reflex in the opposite eye at different sizes. This constructed quadratic relationship is shown by the top line in Figure 8.3. Note that the average of the curve is highly significant.

Superimposed on this line are blue data points derived from altering the size by giving intravenous remifentanil to volunteers. As can be observed, this drug alters the percent light reflex only by changing the size of the pupil, a conclusion demonstrated by other studies (134). The blue points around the regression line all have NPi values above 4.3. The lack of effect of opioids on the light reflex will be discussed further in Chapter 12.

Dividing the top graph of normal reflexes into fractions can provide a number representing the quality of the light reflex. Curves are shown for fractions of 0.8, 0.6, 0.4, and 0.2 of the top normal curve. The fractional curves are then labeled 5, 4, 3, 2, 1, with zero reflex strength on the x-axis. Values for percent reflex and pupil size for each measurement can be viewed on the chart from which the strength of the reflex can be obtained (0 to 5). Algorithms to provide a number on the screen similar to the NPi will very likely be eventually incorporated into most portable pupillometers that measure the light reflex. Each instrument would have a different normal curve depending on the intensity of the light and the duration of the stimulus. The author has tested several portable infrared pupillometers and they have all recorded zero values when measuring metal holes of various diameters.

Comparisons of the new parameter purporting to assess the strength of the light reflex would require studies to compare those numbers to the NPi. Constriction velocity, dilation velocity, and latency numbers can also be retrieved from each light reflex

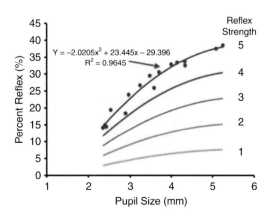

Figure 8.3 The percent light reflex at different pupil sizes documented with the Neuroptics pupillometer. The top curve defines the relationship between percent reflex and pupil size. The blue data points were inserted from a separate study that measured the changes in pupil size brought about by an infusion of remifentanil. This drug alters the light reflex only by altering the size of the pupil. The numbers below 5 are fractions of the top curve and designated lower values indicating a less robust reflex for the size of the pupil during that measurement. Figure constructed by author from data retrieved from 20 consenting volunteers.

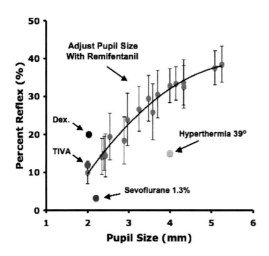

Figure 8.4 Data points are inserted to show the effects of TIVA, vapor anesthetics and hyperthermia on the quality of the light reflex. The points labeled "TIVA" and "Sevoflurane" are extracted from Shirozu et al. (135). Each point represents the average of 10 subjects. The point labeled "Dex" (dexmedetomidine) is from a study of eight subjects who were receiving an anesthetic of propofol and fentanyl. Original drawing by author from data derived from published manuscripts.

measurement. Except for latency, these parameters are also dependent on the initial diameter. In addition to the curves that were constructed using remifentanil, there are other methods of constricting the pupil. Pilocarpine eye drops and near fixation can also constrict the pupil. The curves constructed using these methods are nearly identical to those obtained using opioids and light to change pupil size.

8.4 Effect of Anesthetic Agents

Use of the graph shown in Figure 8.3 allows one to assess the effect of anesthetic and sedative drugs on the quality of the light reflex. Shirozu et al. examined the pupil size and percent reflex changes during the administration of four anesthetic techniques (135). Surgical levels of anesthesia did not depress the reflex during a total intravenous anesthetic (TIVA) with propofol and remifentanil (Figure 8.4). The addition of the vapor anesthetics desflurane and sevoflurane decreased the reflex into the lower ranges (Figure 8.4).

Another study demonstrated that the addition of the NMDA antagonists ketamine and nitrous oxide to 1 percent isoflurane will depress the light reflex. The effect of ketamine on the light reflex in the absence of anesthesia has not been studied, but 70 percent nitrous oxide alone depresses the reflex by 15 percent (136). Importantly, the pupillary light reflex is not abolished during routine surgical levels of anesthesia with any of these agents when using the two pupillometers discussed here. Although nitrous oxide in combination with propofol is less used today, it has been shown that obliteration of the pupillary light reflex will predict absence of movement when very high concentrations of propofol are combined with 60 percent nitrous oxide (137).

8.5 Effect of Nociception on the Pupillary Light Reflex

A study from 1993 demonstrated that noxious stimulation during anesthesia depressed the pupillary light reflex (18). The light reflex recovered when the stimulus was turned

Case Report 8.1

A 45-year-old male was operated on for removal of the sigmoid colon. A thoracic epidural was placed and was used during the case to prevent nociception arising from the surgical dissection. Hypnosis was provided by a continuous infusion of propofol and muscle relaxation was provided by intermittent injections of rocuronium. Prior to closure, the surgeon reached into the upper abdomen to search for a missing sponge. This maneuver stimulated the upper cervical nerves which were not blocked by the epidural. Heart rate and blood pressure increased, and the pupils dilated. The pupillary light reflex was nearly totally blocked during the nociceptive stimulus (Figure 8.5A). Seventy-five micrograms of intravenous fentanyl were given and the pupil constricted slightly and displayed the unusual light reflex waveform shown in Figure 8.5B. Five minutes later, the pupil had constricted to the basal diameter and displayed the reflex shown in Figure 8.5C.

off. As discussed in the previous chapter, this block of the reflex is brought about by increased inhibitory activity at the EW nucleus. Case Report 8.1 illustrates the alteration of the PLR by nociception during general anesthesia.

This case report also illustrates the unique waveform of the pupillary light reflex that can be observed during general anesthesia. Sympathetic tone is lacking during anesthesia so the waveform should be expected to have a delayed re-dilation. Figure 8.5B illustrates this unusual reflex that Loewenfeld called the "Neurotonic" reflex (39). However, when the pupil is maximally constricted after opioids have blocked inhibitory tone, the wave form appears to be solely the result of adding and releasing the excitation of the sphincter by light (Figure 8.5C). Figure 8.5 illustrates the difference in the waveform between the dilated and the constricted pupil during anesthesia.

The result of noxious stimulation on the pupillary light reflex is different in awake subjects as compared to patients who are anesthetized. Guglielminotti et al. studied the changes in the pupillary light reflexes in awake parturients in labor (138). The nociceptive stimulus was the intermittent pains associated with labor contractions. Elevated VAS scores from 0.9 to 7.4 did not block the light reflex as the pupil dilated 21 percent from baseline. During the wakeful state, pupillary dilation is sympathetically mediated and is not significantly affected by inhibition of the EW nucleus. These studies support the conclusions from feline experiments showing that activation of the dilator muscle does not depress the pupillary light reflex (39).

The mechanism of how profound stressful events depress the light reflex in awake humans is unknown and would be difficult to study. With asphyxia, it is very likely that the light reflex is depressed through increased inhibition of the EW nucleus. Topical phenylephrine can depress the light reflex, but that observation is only relevant when the alpha 1 receptors are fully occupied. The report that experimental activation of the dilator muscle in awake animals does not depress the light reflex (13) suggests that the observations by J. Mery and Philippe de la Hire (see Chapter 1) were secondary to increased inhibition of the EW nucleus (see Figure 4.1).

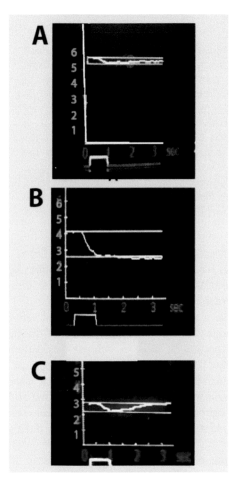

Figure 8.5 A: The light reflex is depressed during nociceptive stimulation during anesthesia. The light stimulus is delivered between the yellow rectangles on each measurement. B: The "neurotonic" pupil as described by Loewenfeld can be observed when the pupil is dilated during general anesthesia with propofol. C: The light reflex of the constricted pupil does not show the same pattern. The images are taken directly from the screen of the Neuroptics PLR-3000 pupillometer. Measurements were taken from a consenting patient during general anesthesia. Photograph of the Neuroptics pupillometer screen by author.

The previous discussion refers to the effect of nociception on the light reflex in awake humans. Cognitive tasks and fear have been reported to depress the light reflex and these effects are also thought to be mediated by inhibitory influences on the EW nucleus (64, 39).

8.6 Effect of Body Temperature and Neuromuscular Blockade

Important questions pertain to the effect of temperature and neuromuscular blocking agents on the light reflex. Patients with intracranial pathologies are often on mechanical ventilation. Because coughing can increase intracranial pressure, it is sometimes desirable to add neuromuscular blocking agents. If these drugs alter the light reflex, it might confound the evaluation of an evolving neurologic condition. As discussed in the previous section, the use of propofol and opioids together does not change the reflex if an analysis is performed as described in Figure 8.4.

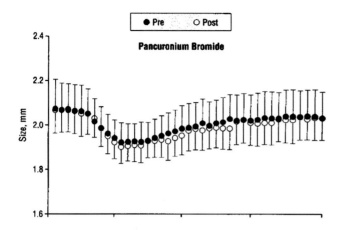

Figure 8.6 Pupillary light reflex measurements after stable levels of general anesthesia were established exhibit no change after pancuronium administration. No alteration of the light reflex was observed. Markers on the x axis are in seconds. Permisssion to reproduce image from *JAMA Neurology*. License Number: 5670890783982.

There is some confusion in the literature relating to the effect of neuromuscular blocking agents on the pupillary light reflex. A popular textbook on coma states that patients with complete paralysis from neuromuscular blocking agents can mimic brain death (12, 139). This is not a trivial issue. Caregivers in emergency rooms might be faced with a resuscitated patient who was intubated with the use of long-acting muscle relaxants. Pupillary measurements are rapid and easy to measure. A dilated pupil with a normal light reflex (see Figure 8.4) might suggest that these patients are awake and paralyzed. Recent reports demonstrate that depolarizing blocking agents such as succinylcholine (15) or nondepolarizing agents such as vecuronium and pancuronium do not block the pupillary light reflex when precise portable pupillometers are used (Figure 8.6; 140).

In routine use, neuromuscular blockers do not enter the CNS or the iris musculature (blood–iris barrier) because the drugs are ionized and fail to pass lipid barriers. With disease states that disrupt the blood–brain barrier, these drugs can then gain access to sites that will produce diminished or absent pupillary reflexes. Some case reports suggest that this can happen with Covid-19 infections and during ECMO circulatory support (141–143). Although there are several infrared pupillometers on the market for purchase (144), the portable instruments as described in Chapter 6 would be ideal to use at the bedside to ascertain if light reflexes are totally absent.

Early studies on the pupillary light reflex and body temperature were initially performed in collaboration with the thermoregulation study group at UCSF. Hypothermia to 35.2 degrees C by itself had little effect on the extent of the light reflex (Figure 8.7; 17), but topical cooling of the eye to below 30 degrees C did alter pupil size, constriction velocity, dilation velocity, and reflex amplitude (145). Patients who survive cold-water immersion are often reported to have nonreactive pupils during resuscitation (146, 147). Muscles become sluggish in cold environments (148), and the iris musculature is no exception (145). For these reasons, the quality of the light reflex during profound induced hypothermia following cardiac arrest should not be relied upon to predict neurologic outcomes (see Chapter 11; 149).

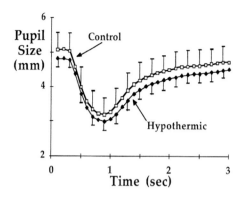

Figure 8.7 Systemic cooling by 1.6°C during anesthesia has no effect on the pupillary light reflex. Permission to reproduce figure from Wolters Kluwer Health, Inc. License Number: 5591970327333.

In awake subjects, induced hyperthermia to 38 degrees C did not alter pupil size or the pupillary light reflex (136). Hyperthermia to 39.4 degrees C during anesthesia dilated the pupil from 2 to above 4 mm and augmented the reflex as measured in mm amplitude (136). However, the percent reflex at 4 mm was only 15 percent. When these values are placed into Figure 8.4, it becomes apparent that the light reflex is depressed by hyperthermia during anesthesia. This presumably comes about by increased inhibition at the EW nucleus brought about by the stress of increased body temperature.

Pupillary Reflex Dilation

If one dips the head of a living cat under water, and exposes its eyes to the rays of the sun, the pupil dilates instead of contracting; however, when exposed in the air to the same rays of the sun, the pupil constricts instead of dilating.

(J. Mery, *Des mouvements de l'iris*, 1704 [32])

9.1 Introduction to PRD and Species Differences

Pupillary reflex dilation (PRD) is the widening of pupillary diameter that occurs following an alerting stimulus, such as a loud sound or a nociceptive stimulus. The survival benefit has never been adequately explained, but may be related to a rapid improvement of vision in dim light. The phenomenon has been studied for over 300 years and provides a rich literature on how pupillary diameter is controlled. During anesthesia, the pupillary dilation following a nociceptive stimulus is more pronounced than the hemodynamic change (Figure 9.1).

There are several species differences and confounding effects of drugs on the extent of PRD. A thorough study of this reflex was summarized by Loewenfeld in 1958 (13), but much has been discovered since that landmark article was published. Infrared pupillometry has revolutionized the study of PRD and consequently has made it a useful measure to quantitate in the anesthetized or heavily sedated patient in the hospital. It is an actively studied parameter of pupillary behavior and it is likely that in the future much will be learned about the practical use of this reflex, and that its use will be expanded to a wider group of physician specialists.

Much of the early work on PRD was performed on anesthetized cats, a species that is exquisitely sensitive to the pupillary dilating effects of circulating catecholamines. A painful stimulus in the anesthetized cat will dilate the pupil even when the sympathetic nerves to the orbit have been severed and the parasympathetic innervation blocked by atropine. In primates, increases of circulating catecholamines have not been shown to dilate the pupil, as has been shown in cats (80). In humans, dramatic elevations of circulating norepinephrine and epinephrine (99, 150–152) fail to produce additional pupillary dilation in anesthetized subjects above that which is observed in the sympathetically blocked pupil. Likewise, the use of vasopressors such as norepinephrine and epinephrine fails to dilate the pupil in anesthetized human subjects. In cats, there is evidence that alpha 2 adrenergic receptors are involved in producing the pupillary reflex dilation after sciatic nerve

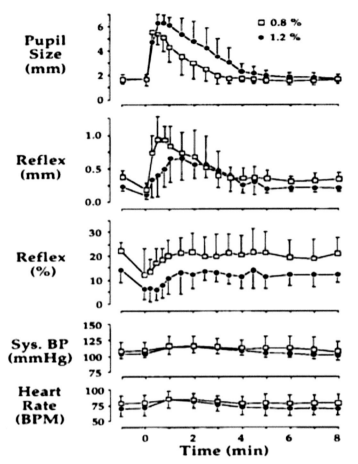

Figure 9.1 Pupillary reflex dilation following tetanic stimulation is a more pronounced reflex than the other autonomic variables such as heart rate and blood pressure. The reflex is more robust at the higher concentration of inhalation anesthetics. Permission for reproduction of image granted by Wolters Kluwer Health, Inc. License Number: 5592521475512.

stimulation, but some other transmitter appears to be involved in these same animals when PRD is produced by stimulation of supraspinal sites (153). It is commonly stated that the locus coeruleus produces inhibition of the EW nucleus (154, 155), but a direct connection has not been established.

It has been shown that dopamine 2 antagonists can block PRD in anesthetized humans, but the actual transmitter for this reflex in humans is not known (89). However, it has been shown that, during anesthesia, PRD is not brought about by activation of the dilator muscle. An analysis of the sympathetic and parasympathetic control of pupil size was performed several years ago by Bonvallet and Zbrozyna (156). These authors observed that during anesthesia a nociceptive stimulus dilated the cat pupil secondary to inhibition of the EW nucleus, whereas when the animals were awakened, the same stimulus produced dilation secondary to activation of the sympathetically innervated dilator muscle (Figure 9.2). Human studies have supported this conclusion (Figure 9.3; 99). There is an exception to this rule: untreated pheochromocytoma can produce massive increases of catecholamines during anesthesia that can produce dilated unreactive pupils (101). Also,

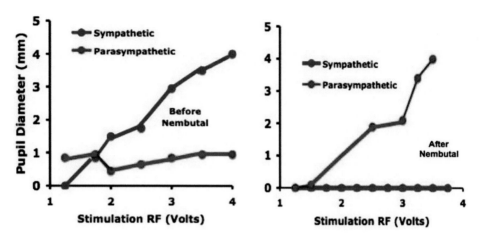

Figure 9.2 This is a reproduction of Figure 6 from the article by Bonvallet and Zbrozyna. In the awake cat, a nociceptive stimulus dilated the pupil secondary to sympathetic activation, whereas during anesthesia, the dilation was produced by inhibition of the EW nucleus. Drawing constructed from the original manuscript.

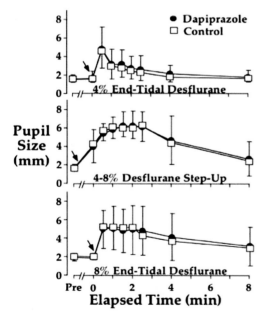

Figure 9.3 PRD is a very robust reflex in anesthetized humans, and it occurs by inhibition of the EW neurons that control pupil size. Blocking the dilator muscle has no effect on the magnitude of the dilation. The inciting stimulus for PRD is nociception, which can arise from a surgical stimulus or from a tetanic electrical stimulus. See Figure 4.1 to locate the site of action and effect of dapiprazole. Permission for reproduction of image granted by Wolters Kluwer Health, Inc. License Number: 5592011105938.

unusual cases of sympathetically mediated pupillary dilation (47) were discussed in Chapter 5 and a case will be presented in Chapter 13. This occurs in patients with Horner's syndrome who have developed denervation hypersensitivity to circulating alpha 1 adrenergic agents such as epinephrine and norepinephrine.

9.2 Ciliospinal Reflex

A common reflex that is often used at the bedside is to pinch the skin over the upper cervical dermatomes and watch for dilation of the ipsilateral pupil (157, 158). This reflex is sometimes used during the neurological examination of comatose patients (12). Jørgensen and Malchow-Møller reported that early return of this reflex after cardiac arrest predicted a favorable neurological outcome (159). Clinicians who find this reflex useful could use the Algiscan pupillometer to accurately record the reflex and document the percentage dilation after each measurement.

The "ciliospinal reflex" is simply another iteration of PRD. When performing the ciliospinal reflex, the noxious stimulus originates from the dermatomes in the upper spinal cord. Reeves and Posner concluded that only an intact spinal cord below the mid cervical level was required to elicit the reflex (160). But the reflex is absent in brain-dead organ donors who have intact sympathetic circulatory reflexes (161). Loewenfeld (39) and others (161) propose that the afferent arm of the reflex extends above the brain stem. The complete sympathetic reflex is thought to traverse a pathway cephalad to the hypothalamus and is therefore not present in brain-dead subjects (39). There is also no evidence that is unilateral. Noxious stimulation of the cervical dermatomes produces dilation of both pupils.

In the anesthetized patient, a noxious stimulus anywhere in the body produces pupillary dilation through inhibition of the EW nucleus (18). Case reports have documented an exaggerated pupillary dilation and pupillary areflexia following generation of the ciliospinal reflex during barbiturate-induced coma (157, 158). Most likely this occurs through inhibition of the EW nucleus and is not produced through activation of the dilator muscle. Inhibitory influences at the EW nucleus can block the pupillary light reflex (see Figure 8.5), as the authors of these reports have observed. It is known that the pupil dilates, and the light reflex is depressed following skin incisions and from noxious stimuli during anesthesia (18, 162).

When performing the ciliospinal reflex, it is useful to know that opioids will depress, and even block, the reflex in both awake and anesthetized subjects. Opioids given to unconscious patients during anesthesia will block the reflex by interfering with the inhibitory action of the nociceptive stimulus on the EW nucleus (Figure 9.4; 134).

As discussed in the previous paragraphs, in awake subjects PRD is brought about primarily by activation of the sympathetic dilator muscle. Aissou et al. studied the effect of morphine on PRD in awake postoperative patients (163). Pain was elicited by pressure on the abdominal wound. The drug depressed the dilation, and the depression was correlated with pain relief. Opioids are known to engage a supraspinal inhibitory effect on nociceptive transmission in the dorsal horn of the spinal cord (164). Presumably, this mechanism accounts for the depression of PRD after opioids in awake subjects. In addition, as the constrictor muscle is activated following opioid administration, the dilator muscle function is simultaneously depressed (see Chapter 10). Therefore, in either awake or anesthetized patients, the ciliospinal reflex will be absent or depressed if opioids have been administered.

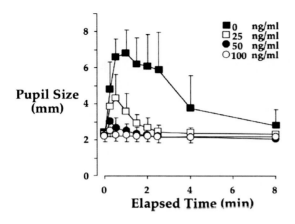

Figure 9.4 Increasing plasma concentrations of alfentanil produce a progressive block of PRD in anesthetized subjects. Permission for reproduction of image granted by Wolters Kluwer Health, Inc. License Number: 5593160241753.

9.3 PRD and Prediction of Movement During Total Intravenous Anesthesia

There are reports that the magnitude of PRD can predict movement when a total anesthetic with propofol and remifentanil is used (165). Accordingly, the analgesic component of a total anesthetic can be measured by quantitating the strength of PRD.

Guglielminotti et al. (166) used the peak dilation after the stimulus of 5 seconds, 50 milliamps to predict movement during dilation of the cervix and uncovered a correlation between PRD and movement. This study was performed in patients receiving total intravenous anesthesia. Studies that examine the relationship between movement and PRD would require a standardized stimulus and some agreed-upon measure of the strength of PRD. This idea might not be suitable for anesthetics conducted with volatile agents because of the enhancement of the reflex by higher concentrations of said agents (18). Examining this relationship during total anesthesia with propofol/remifentanil could have implications on adjusting the dose of opioids to prevent movement in patients that are difficult to manage with pharmacodynamic and computerized infusions alone. The relationship between PRD and movement during total intravenous anesthesia has recently been confirmed by other investigators (167).

A theoretical explanation for the association between movement and pupillary dilation during total intravenous anesthesia has been proposed (167). The EW neurons and the "off cells" in the rostroventral medulla have a similar response to noxious stimulation and to opioids. These two neuronal groups are depressed by nociception, and this depression is blocked by opioids. The "off cells" are spontaneously active during anesthesia and exert an analgesic effect on dorsal horn transmission of nociceptive activity (168, 169). One suggestion is that the EW neurons represent a surrogate measure of "off cell" activity. When the pupil dilates, this coincides with a pause in "off cell" activity, and movement occurs. This is only a theoretical analysis and, without the option of recording neuronal activity in the brain stem, this idea cannot be confirmed.

Palliative sedation at the end of life is often managed with opioids as the primary analgesic agent. Pupillary dilation then suggests a lack of analgesia. Avoidance of arousal is an important aspect of palliative sedation, and a dilated pupil then indicates either inadequate opioid dose or tolerance to opioids. Elyn et al. have presented a case report that demonstrates the value of infrared pupillometry during palliative sedation (170).

9.4 Testing for Local Anesthetic Block During Combined Regional–General Anesthesia

The use of PRD to detect blocked dermatomes during combined regional–general anesthesia is one of the practical uses of this reflex. Nociception brought about by an artificial stimulus will dilate the pupil with a latency of approximately 1 second (171). The technique was originally used to determine the cephalic extent of local anesthetic blockade during combined epidural/general anesthesia (172). Electrical stimulation through electrodes placed over dermatomes that have been rendered analgesic by the epidural injection will not produce any dilation of the pupil (Figure 9.5). Assessment of PRD from the C5 dermatome provides the clinician with a rough estimate of the degree to which epidural opioid injection has resulted in spread into the cervical dermatomes (173).

The idea of testing for unblocked segments during the combined technique is an application of pupillometry that has been suggested by other manuscripts (174, 175, 176). In response to a brief tetanic stimulus, the pupillary response in unblocked dermatomes is rapid and definitive. In contrast, the hemodynamic and EEG responses are delayed and prolonged (137). Because of this feature, the anesthesiologist can test several dermatomes in rapid succession and then decide if further analgesics are required prior to emergence. This idea would require either a moveable stimulating electrode or several electrodes placed in selected areas prior to induction. Awakening a patient undergoing a combined technique with an inadequate sensory block is uncomfortable for them unless opioids have been administered prior to emergence from anesthesia. Direct stimulation of muscles to test for unblocked dermatomes can produce unwanted movements. Electrodes should ideally be placed over bony prominences. If electrodes are stimulated on areas of the skin that cover large muscle groups, then it is advisable to have patients partially paralyzed from prior use of muscle relaxants.

When using PRD to detect unblocked dermatomes, it is important to be aware of other drugs and patient characteristics that can block or enhance PRD. The combined "regional–general" anesthetic method is usually conducted without opioids, but if those

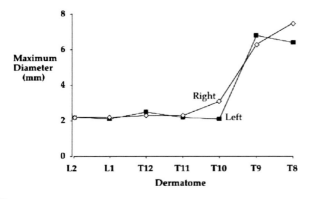

Figure 9.5 Surface-stimulating electrodes were used to measure PRD prior to awakening the patient from general anesthesia. Upon awakening, the epidural block level was located on dermatomes below T10. Permission for reproduction of image granted by Wolters Kluwer Health, Inc. License Number: 5593320575319.

drugs are given in high doses, PRD will be blocked (Figure 9.4; 177). Dopamine 2 antagonists suppress PRD during general anesthesia (89). Other antiemetics such as ondansetron have no effect on PRD. Dexmedetomidine is often used during general anesthesia and has been reported to diminish PRD (Figure 9.6). Nitrous oxide augments pupillary reflex dilation during the stress of a rapid rise in desflurane concentration (Figure 9.7; 150).

Other confounding factors are patients with immobile pupils because of surgery, diabetic neuropathy, or senile miosis. Because these syndromes are rare and dopamine antagonists are not in widespread use today, it is uncommon to note the absence of PRD during general anesthesia unless high-dose opioid therapy is used. Placement of stimulating electrodes on dermatomes innervated by cranial nerves will serve to determine if the pupil will dilate following stimulation of unblocked segments. The epidural block cannot extend above the foramen magnum, so electrodes on the brow or side of the face can serve as control locations. These areas are innervated by the mandibular nerve, so testing on the face for PRD will answer the question of whether factors other than local anesthetic blockade account for the lack of dilation after noxious stimulation.

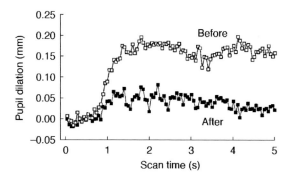

Figure 9.6 Pupillary reflex dilation during general anesthesia before (top) and after (bottom) the intravenous administration of dexmedetomidine. Permission for reproduction of image granted by John Wiley & Sons. License Number: 5593081312611.

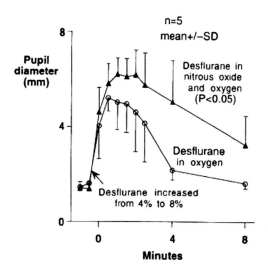

Figure 9.7 A rapid abrupt rise in the concentration of desflurane produces pupillary dilation that is augmented by nitrous oxide. Permission for reproduction of image granted by Wolters Kluwer Health, Inc. License Number: 5604221183079.

The same technique has been used to verify that adequate local anesthetic blockade has been achieved following peripheral nerve injections. With current practice, it is common to place peripheral nerve blocks and then induce general anesthesia prior to the time when the local anesthetic has reached the full extent of sensory loss. Many patients elect to be completely asleep during their operations, but still prefer the additional advantages of peripheral nerve blocks. When general anesthesia is added to peripheral nerve block, one can test for adequacy of the block with pupillometry in a manner like that used during combined epidural–general anesthesia (see Case Report 14.4 in Chapter 14).

Testing with pupillometry allows the anesthesiologist to know the true extent of the block before the incision is made. Clearly, if pupillometry reveals the block to be inadequate, an alternative plan to provide analgesia may be required for the anticipated procedure. Some would argue that the adequacy of the peripheral nerve block can be ascertained by the heart rate or blood pressure response to the skin incision. However, beta-adrenergic blockers or opioids given during the induction of general anesthesia can obtund the hemodynamic response to skin incision, whereas pupillometry can detect small dilations even after these drugs have been given.

There are other instances where the surgeon might prefer to inject peripheral nerves just before emergence. Gentle pressure on the surgical wound during closure will dilate the pupil if the area is not blocked by the local anesthetic. This is an easy technique that can be applied to any case of a combined "regional–general" anesthetic.

In the pediatric population, it is common to perform a caudal injection of local anesthetics or inject peripheral nerves during general anesthesia (175). Pupillometry in these cases would be a method of assuring an adequate block before emergence. Very little can be learned about the amount of pain experienced from a crying infant in the recovery room. However, pupillometric evidence of analgesia surrounding the surgical site before emergence from general anesthesia would eliminate pain as a significant factor contributing to the unpleasant feelings of a crying baby (Figure 9.8).

The idea of using a nerve stimulator to test for blocked and unblocked dermatomes might be cumbersome without an instrument that is designed specifically for that purpose. The AlgiScan pupillometer made in Marseille, France, is a portable infrared pupillometer that is especially designed to provide a standardized noxious stimulus to the skin of anesthetized patients. The resulting pupillary dilation that is observed on the screen of the pupillometer provides a measure of opioid effect and to detect the extent of regional anesthetics. Figure 6.7 illustrates how a cable will attach the pupillometer electrodes for stimulation of selected dermatomes. The pupil will dilate if the dermatomal segments are not blocked by the regional block.

9.5 Pupillometry Using PRD and Nociception Monitors

9.5.1 Nociception During Anesthesia

Today, there are several nociception monitors available that are designed to measure nociception during anesthesia. The NOL (Nociception Level) monitor gathers data from a finger probe that records skin temperature, photoplethysmography, accelerometry, and galvanic skin response. There are conflicting views on whether this monitor can improve the care of the anesthetized patient. The Analgesia Nociception Index (ANI) monitor

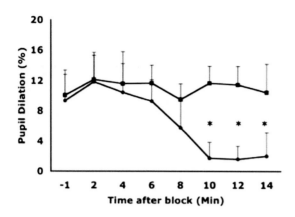

Figure 9.8 Stimulation with surface electrodes at L4 and C5 after caudal injection of local anesthetic in an infant. Note that PRD in the lumbar dermatome is slowly diminished, but the PRD from stimulation of the C5 dermatome is unaffected. Permission for reproduction of image granted by Wolters Kluwer Health, Inc. License Number: 5593321438493.

takes data from the heart rate variability and provides a scale from 1 to 100 indicating the degree of nociception. The surgical pleth index (SPI) derives a number from 0 to 100 that is calculated from the pulse-wave amplitude and the RR interval from the electrocardiogram.

One drawback of these monitors is that they cannot predict how a patient will respond to a future noxious stimulus. For example, these monitors typically reveal low values in the interval between induction and the skin incision. This occurs simply because there is no ongoing nociception prior to surgery. But the most intense nociceptive stimulus in many surgical procedures is the initial skin incision. Thus, one important issue is anticipating how the patient will respond to this very intense initial stimulus.

It is generally accepted that an analysis of the EEG cannot always accurately predict the degree of nociception during anesthesia. Monitors that measure hypnosis and sedation take information from the EEG and process it into a number that is said to measure lack of awareness. But hypnosis or loss of awareness with these devices measures cortical waveforms that typically derive limited information from deep in the brain stem and spinal cord, where nociception can give rise to reflex movements and other autonomic responses that characterize the stress response (134). The EEG response to nociceptive stimulation can be detected, but it is less robust than the response from the pupil and has a comparatively delayed onset (137).

PRD is a brain stem reflex and theoretically might provide information regarding the nociception–antinociception balance. With an anesthetic that uses opioids for analgesia, pupillometry can provide an assessment of opioid effect prior to the incision (178). The AlgiScan device incorporates an algorithm that stimulates with low-intensity electrical tetanic current and then detects the change in pupil diameter that is produced by the stimulus. This method of detecting opioid effect in anesthetized subjects is called the Pupillary Pain Index (PPI) and is graded on a scale of 0–6 (179). This mode of stimulation can be delivered prior to the incision. Because it is a mild stimulus, it does not produce unwanted movement or changes in hemodynamics.

With an anesthetic that uses opioids for analgesia, detection of opioid effect can be tested with appropriate settings on portable pupillometers. It could be a useful tool to predict the nociceptive response to the more intense stimulus brought about by the skin incision (180). An important topic of discussion is whether depression of PRD is a measurement of antinociception or whether it is a measurement of opioid effect. Further studies are required to detect whether depression of PRD is observed during anesthetics that rely on non-opioid intraoperative analgesics. Some studies have suggested that the PPI predicts the behavioral response to tracheal tube suctioning in comatose patients (181). The PPI has been suggested as a useful measurement to predict pain on emergence from anesthesia in children (179). Others have studied the PPI to predict neurologic outcomes after cardiac arrest (182).

9.5.2 Pupillometry and Pain

In an awake subject, pain is a subjective experience that only the patient can describe. Attempts to measure pain objectively sometimes rely on autonomic changes such as heart rate, blood pressure, sweating, and pupillary dilation. Nociception as defined by Sherrington over 100 years ago refers to the physiological responses to activation of specific nerve endings that respond to noxious stimuli and were designated nociceptors (36). The response to activation of nociceptors in awake subjects is variable, so the same degree of nociception can produce severe pain in one subject, but minimal pain in another subject. As discussed in the previous section on PRD, it is possible to detect nociception in anesthetized patients, and this technique is useful in detecting blocked and unblocked dermatomes during general anesthesia. But nociception and pain are different entities. Nociception during anesthesia is not painful simply because the patient is not awake. The idea of an objective measure of pain might be a useful addition to the management of uncommunicating patients or those with opioid abuse disorders. These patients can often request opioid therapy without an obvious source of nociception. On the other hand, there are patients who have pain, but deny it because they are opposed to drug treatments of any kind.

Although Aissou et al. used pupillary dilation to titrate opioids in the recovery room (163), it is unlikely that steady unrelenting pain can be objectively measured with pupillometry. The pupillary dilation that is observed following activation of nociceptors is an abrupt change. It is not sustained if the stimulation continues. Sustained activation of nociceptors can therefore produce a transient dilation of the pupil that dissipates even though the experience of pain continues. Some measures derived from portable pupillometers might be used to measure intermittent acute pain (183–184). However, pupillometry does not accurately measure unrelenting pain such as is observed in the emergency room (185). Chapter 12 has a further discussion of the relationship between the effect of opioids on the pupil and how those measures correlate with pain scores.

Chapter 10

Measuring Inhibition at the EW Nucleus

> He plumed the deepness of her ever-varying pupils, with their radiating
> fibrils of blue, and black, and gray, and violet.

(Thomas Hardy, *Tess of the d'Urbervilles*)

The EW nucleus has both excitatory and inhibitory afferent inputs. Most of the current practical use of portable pupillometry is directed toward assessment of the strength of the excitatory activation of the sphincter muscle of the iris, hence the algorithms such as the NPi and the QPi discussed in Chapter 8. But inhibition of the EW nucleus can also be measured and can provide useful information to the clinician. Inhibition of the EW nucleus during general anesthesia was discussed in the previous chapter. Two simple methods can be used in awake subjects to gauge the strength of the inhibitory influence on the EW nucleus, pupillary unrest in ambient light (PUAL), and the "light off" (LO) reflex.

10.1 Pupillary Unrest in Ambient Light

In normal ambient light, the pupil fluctuates in size. These changes in pupil size have been termed pupillary unrest in ambient light (PUAL). This term is used to identify it as a different phenomenon from what has traditionally been termed hippus, or PUI, as will be discussed in the next section.

In the awake state, PUAL is observed by looking closely at the pupil of a friend or by using an electronic pupillometer that precisely records pupil size. It is absent in the dark because excitation is lacking. It is absent after large doses of opioids or during general anesthesia because inhibition is lacking. Animal studies are of little value in the determination of how PUAL is generated in humans. For example, the wide fluctuations in pupil size that are observed in rats during anesthesia (186) are not observed in humans using conventional methods. Anesthetics and opioids have variable actions on the EW nucleus depending on the species (187). In humans, opioids block the inhibitory influences of nociception and awareness on the EW nucleus (56). In a later chapter, the value of PUAL in the assessment of opioid effect will be discussed.

PUAL is a chaotic variation not linked to any stimulus such as changes in light level, noxious stimulation, cognitive effort, or alerting stimuli. It has been observed for several decades that changes in cognition or arousing stimuli can dilate the pupil. Similarly, an abrupt painful stimulus will produce a startle reflex and produce pupillary dilation. Muscular activity, such as a voluntary deep breath, produces pupillary dilation. These various stimuli and mental activities can all produce changes in pupil size, but are unrelated to PUAL, which is the simply the variability of pupil size that is brought

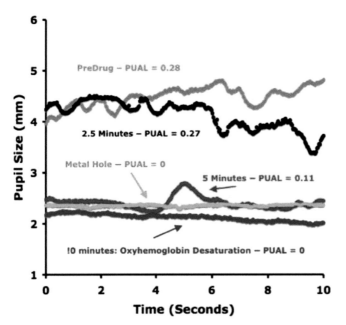

Figure 10.1 The green tracing is taken on a metal hole of 2.3 mm in diameter. Note the presence of pupillary fluctuations in the top two tracings taken from this awake patient. This patient was given an overdose of remifentanil and the pupillary fluctuations diminished to zero (blue tracing), like that observed when taking a measurement from a metal hole (green tracing). Permission for reproduction of image was granted from Elsevier under the terms of the Creative Commons CC BY License, which permits unrestricted use in any medium.

about by the normal state of wakefulness in the presence of a steady light source. Lacking either wakefulness or light, the pupil is not fluctuating and then PUAL is the same value as that obtained by measuring metal holes of fixed diameters (Figure 10.1). PUAL values have been reported to range from 0.1 to 0.8 arbitrary units (AUs) and this large spread reflects the various methods that have been used to process the signal. Mean values cannot be compared between publications because of these differences. If the same algorithm is used, then the PUAL values vary with age and use of opioids (188, 189). In addition, the Neuroptics PLR-3000 and Algiscan sample at different rates, so the values of PUAL are very slightly different, but the response to opioids is the same. Please note that some patients can be awake, but not aware. Our preliminary observations indicate that an awake patient who is not aware can have normal PUAL values.

As demonstrated by Stark (190), the fluctuations in pupil size are equal in both eyes (Figure 10.2). This equality of PUAL in both eyes implies that there is a common source that generates a variable input to the pupillary sphincter (190). It is generally accepted that the source of the size fluctuations that produce PUAL resides in the EW nucleus (191). The sphincter muscle of the iris then fluctuates as it is driven by this nucleus. Sympathetic innervation can alter the magnitude of the fluctuation by exerting a pull on the dilator muscle, but the frequency of the fluctuation does not change (Figure 10.3).

The interplay that takes place between excitation and inhibition produces the fluctuation called PUAL (Figure 10.4). Excessive light above 500 lux will result in a tight miosis, and then PUAL begins to decline (Figure 10.5; 188). PUAL declines to near zero during loss of consciousness during propofol anesthesia (Figures 10.6 and 10.7).

For reasons not understood, functional integrity of the midbrain sites that allow the awake state are a necessary factor in the generation of PUAL. For example, it is known that nociceptive stimulation that arises during general anesthesia inhibits the EW nucleus and dilates the pupil, but it does not elicit PUAL (Figure 10.6). Presumably,

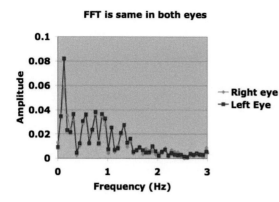

Figure 10.2 Two pupillometers are synchronized and the Fast Fourier Transform is used to show the frequency/amplitude characteristics of each eye. Note that the fluctuations are the same in both eyes. Pupillometer tracings taken from consenting volunteer subject.

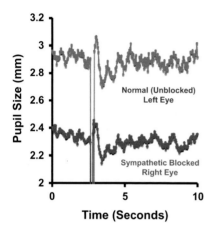

Figure 10.3 Blocking the dilator muscle of the iris with brimonidine decreases pupillary unrest amplitudes, but does not alter the frequency of fluctuations. Pupillometer tracings taken from a consenting volunteer subject.

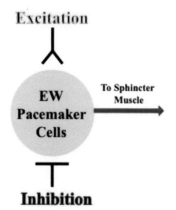

Figure 10.4 Competing excitatory and inhibitory inputs into the EW nucleus generate PUAL. When both inhibition and excitation are blocked, the EW neurons fire at a rapid pace, resulting in the miosis of sleep. Permission to reproduce image granted from Elsevier under License Number 5594871016438.

the inhibitory source during general anesthesia has different features compared to the inhibition that is present during the awake state (see previous discussion, Chapter 9).

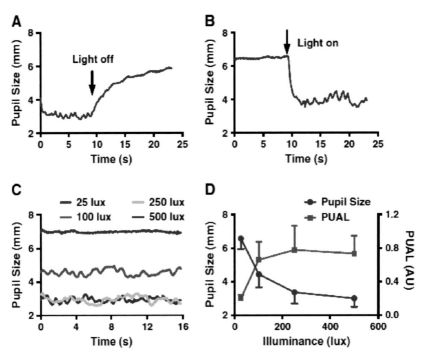

Figure 10.5 Pupillary unrest requires light (A and B) and a source of inhibition at the EW nucleus. In darkness, PUAL is absent (A, B, and C), but it is present in normal ambient light conditions. However, when the ambient light exceeds approximately 500 lux, then pupillary unrest gradually diminishes (D). Permission to reproduce image obtained from Elsevier under License Number 5592530266157.

The infrared portable pupillometers can record the small alterations in pupil size that occur in ambient light. Intuitively, it might seem unlikely that a hand-held instrument could record these small fluctuations of the pupil in an awake subject whose eyes might move slightly within the orbit during the measurement. To convince the clinician that this is possible, it has been shown that fixed apertures can be measured with these instruments, and they show essentially no fluctuations in size (Figure 10.1). With practice, it becomes easy to display the pupil size over a 10-second measurement. The measurement is taken with the non-measured eye covered by the operator's hand. The measured eye is illuminated by a source of light in the pupillometer that is equivalent to average indoor lighting. More detailed descriptions of the measurement technique have been published (188, 189).

The problem then arises as to how to place a number on the frequency and the amplitude of the pupil size changes that are observed. Quantitation of fluctuations is performed using a Fast Fourier Transform (FFT) that graphs the amplitude of fluctuations against the frequency of fluctuation. The value of each measurement is then obtained by calculating the area under the curve of the FFT. This value is called PUAL and is given values in arbitrary units. Some of the commercial portable pupillometers provide an automatic readout of PUAL after each measurement.

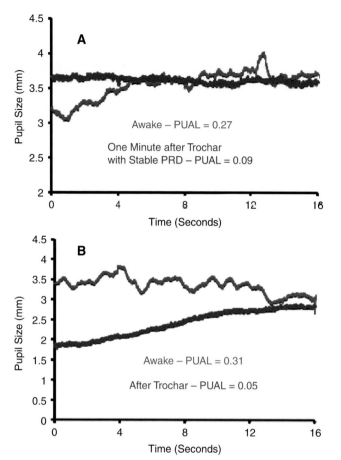

Figure 10.6 A and B: During general anesthesia, the fluctuations of the pupil that produce PUAL are absent. Dilation of the pupil by nociception during anesthesia does not produce the same fluctuations (PUAL) that can be observed in the awake state (220). Permission to reproduce image obtained from Springer Nature under License Number 5627770361301.

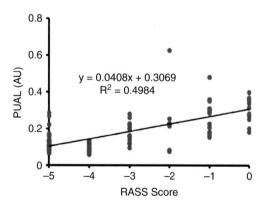

Figure 10.7 An infusion of propofol leads to a loss of PUAL as unconsciousness intervenes, at which time PUAL is absent. RASS: Richmond Agitation–Sedation Scale, a measure of sedation or agitation. Minus 5 is unarousable sedation. Permission to reproduce image obtained from Springer Nature under License Number 5627770361301.

The fluctuations of the pupil in ambient light occur primarily in frequencies between 0.1 Hz and 5 Hz, so the area below the curve that calculates PUAL is typically between the frequencies of 0.3 and 3 Hz. The pupil is unable to oscillate at high frequencies because pupillary movements are generated by activation of sluggish smooth muscles.

PUAL varies within the same subject about 30 percent from trial to trial (188, 189). There are several factors that contribute to this variability and understanding them will allow the operator to have more consistent measurements. Ideally, a 10-second measurement would not have large (1 mm) slow changes in diameter. Distractions during the measurement such as extraneous conversations, loud banging noises, voluntary deep breaths, questions directed to the patient, and extraneous lighting changes can all contribute to these large shifts in the baseline. Patients in opioid withdrawal will also exhibit these large swings in the baseline diameter, which occur even without an inciting stimulus to provoke the dilation. When these artifacts appear in the tracing, it becomes impossible to perform the FFT and a repeat measurement is indicated. Patients typically do not object to this test and a proper measurement will provide much more useful information than one that has artifacts.

The ability of the portable instruments to record the pupillary fluctuations is made possible by algorithms within the instrument that track the aperture even during hand movements or movement of the aperture. Eye blinking is similarly treated with the use of extrapolations (Figure 10.8). It should be noted that a prolonged eye closure that is more than the upper limit of typical blink (0.4 seconds) would be followed by either a small dilation or a small constriction of the pupil depending on the intensity of the ambient light that illuminates the pupil. It is more appropriate to label these as long duration eye closures, rather than true blinks, and then eliminate them from consideration as a true measure of PUAL. Eye closures can be minimized by proper instructions to the patient before the measurements are taken.

10.2 Pupil Diameter Changes Unrelated to PUAL

Research on the pupil has provided a unique approach to the detection of sleepiness and is accomplished by measuring pupil size in darkness for 5 minutes. In awake subjects, the pupil will be large and stable in size. As drowsiness develops, the inhibitory influences that arise from the awareness centers of the brain begin to intermittently wane. An exaggerated form of pupillary fluctuations, called hippus, then develops. Prolonged recordings of pupil size of a tired subject will show intermittent pupillary constriction, then brisk re-dilations. The constrictions are related to intermittent failure of inhibitory tone. Eventually, the tired subject will fall asleep and then the inhibitions are lost. The pupil then constricts to the small diameter of the sleeping subject. On the other hand, an alert subject will show a more smoothed stable pupil size recording. These waves can then be calibrated and quantitated for each individual subject and serve as a measure of sleepiness. This measure has been labeled the Pupillary Unrest Index (PUI) (192).

Excessive tiredness is known to diminish the capacity to concentrate and carry out demanding tasks. It is therefore useful to know when any one individual is partially incapacitated from lack of sleep. Airline pilots, anesthesiologists, truck drivers, physician residents, registered nurses, and surgeons are often required to work extended hours without any meaningful rest periods. Society demands competency from persons whose expert judgement is essential to the well-being of large numbers of the population. The PUI has been proposed as a marker for excessive tiredness (192–196), but it requires at least 5 minutes to complete and is unsuitable for routine clinical work. Neuroptics sells desktop pupillometers with head mounts that can evaluate sleepiness with long duration measurements. There are no reports of using portable instruments to measure the PUI.

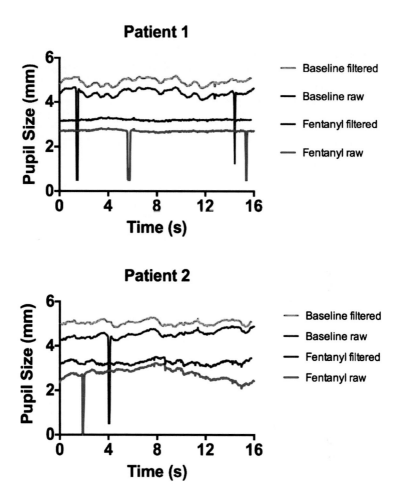

Figure 10.8 An accurate measure of PUAL requires that an algorithm is used to remove baseline drift and artifacts caused by blinks. Pupillometer tracings taken from consenting volunteer subjects.

The Neuroptics PLR-3000 will record pupil size for up to 10 minutes, but whether this long duration measurement in darkness would identify tiredness has not been studied.

This book would not be complete if it did not discuss the Adaptive Gain Theory presented by Aston-Jones and Cohen in 2005 (197). This theory proposed that the neuronal firing patterns of the locus coeruleus (LC) neurons were associated with different behavioral patterns. Phasic LC activity was thought to be related to performance of tasks, whereas tonic LC activity was associated with disengagement from current tasks. Investigators later reported that tonic LC activity enhanced the gain of sensory inputs and was associated with an increase in the size of the pupil (198).

The pupil size changes reported by these authors occur on a different time scale compared to those retrieved during measurement of PUAL. Portable pupillometers could be programmed for long duration measurements that might be relevant for detecting these task-related behaviors. Regarding the low frequencies, it has been reported that the fluctuations of the pupil below 0.1 Hz are amplified during meditation (199). In the clinical setting, it is cumbersome to record these low frequencies because they require a relatively long period of measurement time. For example, a fluctuation at 0.1 Hz requires 10 seconds for just one cycle. To evaluate the power at these low frequencies requires up to 2 minutes of recording time and would not be convenient for clinical use.

10.3 Light Off (LO) Reflex

The "light off" (LO) reflex is a reflex that is easy to measure, but has been neglected in the scientific literature. The LO reflex is different from the pupillary light reflex. The "light on" reflex is brought about by an increase in tension of the sphincter muscle through activation of the EW nucleus by light. The LO reflex, on the other hand, is brought about by inhibition of the EW nucleus and an increase in tone of the dilator muscle. Because of these differences, the LO reflex has information that the pupillary (light on) reflex does not provide. This reflex has been studied in volunteers, but has not been extensively studied in patients. Omary et al. used the LO reflex to study patients with Horner's syndrome because it is thought to be partially generated by increased tension in the dilator muscle (81).

The pupillary LO reflex is produced when white light is directed into the pupil and then abruptly turned off. The reflex has been studied for several decades (39). An understanding of the central mechanism of the early phase of the LO reflex might have potential clinical value. When white light is turned off and both eyes are in darkness, the pupil begins to dilate within 300–500 milliseconds. The dilation continues rapidly at first and then more slowly for several minutes. The final dark-adapted pupil size is not achieved until retinal receptors have adjusted to the new dark environment. A typical analysis is based on measurements taken when the intensity of the initial white light is set to between 350 and 500 lux.

The LO reflex is illustrated in Figure 10.9 (blue line). It is apparent that the pupillary LO reflex has a different time course than the "light on" (red line) reflex. The rapid onset

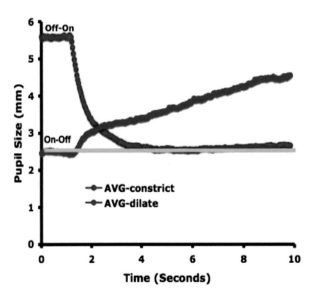

Figure 10.9 The light on reflex shown in red is rapid in onset and is completed within 4 seconds. A longer duration measurement would typically show pupillary escape as described in Chapter 8. The light off reflex shown in blue is delayed and is not completed at 10 seconds. Pupillary measurements taken from a consenting volunteer.

pupillary light on reflex (red line) has a relatively short latency and reaches a maximum response early (4 seconds). The LO reflex has a longer latency and is slow to develop. The response is not complete until several minutes have passed after the light is turned off. Observe that the pupil size after 10 seconds has not yet reached the initial pupil size of the dark-adapted pupil (red tracing). The prolonged time course of dark adaption is due to the slow process of rhodopsin generation that takes nearly 30 minutes. The early pupillary dilation occurs more quickly and is the subject of the "light off" response discussed in this book.

A consistent technique to measure the LO reflex is required to make this reflex useful. If the LO duration is close to 1 minute, then the end diameter minus the start diameter will be the same as the (light on) pupillary light reflex when measured in darkness. In other words, at LO, the pupil will dilate up to the dark diameter that would be observed in total darkness and the LO amplitude will equal the extent of the pupillary light reflex. This is just another way of saying that after a light stimulus, the dark diameter pupil constricts a certain number of mm, and if the measurement continues long enough, it will dilate the same number of mm back to the original diameter prior to light on.

For the busy clinician, it is time-consuming to retrieve information that requires long duration pupillary measurements. One method to circumvent this problem is to direct light into the measured eye and program the instrument to turn the light off after 1 second and then measure the pupil diameter for the following 9 seconds. This technique measures the re-dilation of the light reflex in more detail as compared to the dilation velocity that is recorded following the standard light reflex. A standard technique is essential if this measure is to be trended over time.

The difference between light on and the light off reflexes relates to the type of neurotransmitter receptors and ion channels that mediate each response. The pupillary light reflex is presumably mediated through rapidly acting gated ion channels that are characterized by receptors and ion channels that are different domains of the same protein. On the other hand, the LO response is slow to develop. These slow-onset responses are characteristic of G-protein receptors that entail the activation of slower second messenger enzymes located in the cytoplasm. The previously discussed post illumination pupillary constriction (60, 61) is not apparent when white light is the illuminating source.

The LO reflex in awake subjects is discussed first and will then be compared to the LO reflex in the anesthetized subject. The awake and asleep LO reflexes are different.

10.4 LO Reflex: Awake Subjects

At any one moment, there are hundreds of simultaneous active excitatory and inhibitory synapses on a single neuron in the central nervous system (Figure 10.10; 200). The excitatory/inhibitory (E/I) balance determines the rate of firing of those neurons. In the case of the neurons in the EW nucleus, an increase in ambient light will favor the excitatory input to the EW neurons and the pupil will constrict. This is the pupillary light reflex. On the other hand, an abrupt change from light to dark will alter the E/I balance in favor of inhibition and the pupil will dilate. This change in pupil size represents the early phase of dark adaption and occurs prior to any change in the sensitivity of the retina that relies on the generation of rhodopsin.

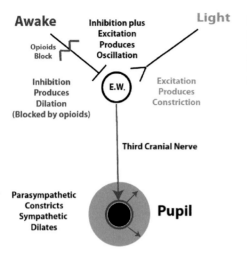

Figure 10.10 Inhibition and excitation of the EW nucleus are both active and contribute to the size of the pupil. Permission to reproduce this image was granted by Elsevier under the terms of the Creative Commons CC BY License, which permits unrestricted use in any medium.

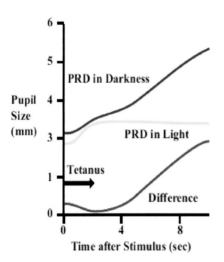

Figure 10.11 A bright light directed into the non-measured eye blocks the inhibitory dilation of the pupil brought about by a noxious stimulus in an anesthetized volunteer. Permission to reproduce this image was obtained from Wolters Kluwer Health, Inc., under License Number 5592040057072.

The light off reflex is not the same reflex as pupillary reflex dilation (PRD) that was discussed in Chapter 9. Unlike PRD, it is not an arousal response, but rather it is the early pupillary response that begins the process of improving vision in darkness.

With the awake subject in ambient light, both the excitatory and inhibitory influences are directed into the EW nucleus. Excitation and inhibition compete at the EW nucleus to determine the firing rate of these neurons. Figure 10.11 illustrates, for example, how a bright light directed into the contralateral pupil can nearly eliminate the pupillary dilation brought about by an intense nociceptive stimulus that inhibits the nucleus (201). The interaction is shown at the arrow in Figure 10.12, whereby excitation and inhibition compete with each other at the EW nucleus. The action of light excitation to overcome the inhibition of the EW nucleus is a common occurrence that can be readily

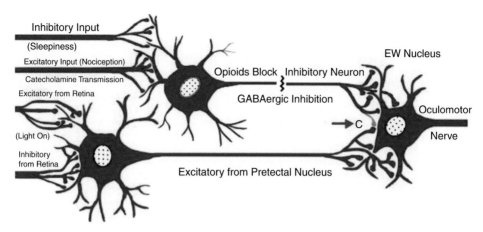

Figure 10.12 Excitation and inhibition are simultaneously active in the awake subject in ambient light. Excitation and inhibition compete (C) for control of EW firing rate (at the red arrow). Opioids block the effect of inhibition on the EW nucleus. Permission for reproduction of image was granted from Elsevier under the terms of the Creative Commons CC BY License, which permits unrestricted use in any medium.

observed by measuring pupil size while an awake subject (inhibition is active) is exposed to bright daylight. And, as has been previously discussed, an intense acute nociceptive stimulus during anesthesia that produces inhibition at the EW nucleus will dilate the pupil and briefly attenuate the light reflex (Figure 8.5; 18).

The inhibitory input into the EW nucleus arises from the arousal nuclei within the mesencephalic reticular formation located below the third nerve nucleus (Figure 10.13). These arousal nuclei include the locus coeruleus, pedunculopontine tegmental nucleus, the mesopontine tegmental nucleus portions of the raphe nucleus, and the dopamine tegmental nuclei (202). An orexin pathway from the posterior hypothalamus activates the arousal nuclei and adds additional inhibition of the EW nucleus. The influence of the recently described mesopontine tegmental anesthesia area on the EW nucleus is unclear (203).

The exact pathways and transmitters involved in producing inhibition at the EW nucleus in humans are unknown, although many theories have been presented. Many authors have written about the direct connection between the locus coeruleus and the EW nucleus with the assumption that the inhibitory transmitter at the EW nucleus is an alpha 2 adrenergic inhibitory process (154, 155, 204). Not all studies have concluded that the locus coeruleus is the primary source of inhibition (205). There is also no evidence that the alpha 2 adrenergic receptor is activated during inhibition of the locus coeruleus in rabbits (206). The evidence for alpha 2 adrenergic inhibitory transmission at the locus coeruleus in humans is not yet complete. Many studies have been performed on species that have different responses to drugs as compared to humans (207). The canine preparation has many pharmacological similarities to humans regarding effect of drugs on pupil size and pupillary reactivity. Opioids, for example, constrict the dog pupil just as with humans, although the dose required is much larger compared to that required for humans. In dogs, direct application of acetylcholine analogues in the proximity of the EW nucleus inhibits the nucleus via a muscarinic mechanism (20, 208).

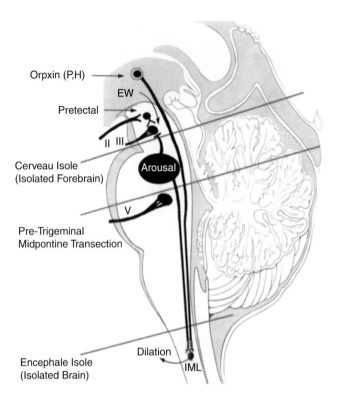

Figure 10.13 A sagittal view of the brain stem that illustrates the position of the arousal nuclei in the upper mesencephalon that dilate the pupil and promote the awake state. EW: Edinger Westphal nucleus. IML: Intermediolateral Nucleus. Drawing by Ping Hill, Research Intern, University of California, San Francisco.

Electrolytic lesions in the area below the third nerve permit surgical procedures on cats without anesthesia (5, 8, 209). Bremer characterized the appearance of cats with these lesions in his classic discussion of the *cerveau isole* (see Figure 10.13 and further discussion in the Preface; 6). The EEG displays the slow-wave high-amplitude pattern of sleep, and the pupils are constricted. Light reflexes were present, but the pupils did not dilate following stimulation via the olfactory nerves. Moreover, applications of strychnine onto the cortical surface changed the EEG sleeping pattern, but did not dilate the pupil (6). Other later classical papers revealed that transection across the mid pons just rostral to the fifth cranial nerve resulted in a pupil that was mid position and responded with dilation following olfactory stimulation (210). Within the past 30 years, studies have demonstrated that between the two transactions there are the potent arousal systems that activate the EEG and dilate the pupil (202).

The LO dilation is brought about through a combination of inhibition of the EW nucleus and an increase in tone of the dilator muscle. Figure 10.14 demonstrates that if the dilator tone is increased by topical application of dilute phenylephrine, then the LO dilation is more robust. Alternatively, if the dilator tone is weakened by topical application of brimonidine, then the LO response is diminished. Loewenfeld has reported that severing the postganglionic sympathetic nerves that innervate the dilator muscle does not block the reflex, but does attenuate it (39).

The role of the sympathetic dilator muscle is partially related to the dual innervation of the parasympathetic portion of the ciliary nerve that sends projections to the sphincter

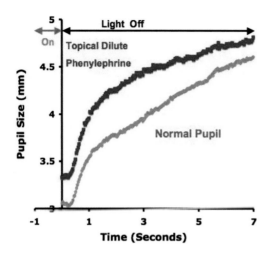

Figure 10.14 Topical application of phenylephrine augments the LO reflex. Pupillary measurements taken from a consenting volunteer subject.

as well as the dilator. When the sphincter is activated by light and opioid therapy, the dilator muscle is simultaneously inhibited (Figure 10.15; 211, 212). When the light is turned off, the excitation of the sphincter is removed. Simultaneously, inhibition of the dilator is lost and this muscle can then progressively pull on the weakened sphincter to dilate the pupil.

10.5 LO During Anesthesia and after Opioids

The LO reflex in anesthetized subjects is different from the same reflex in awake subjects. During most anesthetics, it is common to use opioids to blunt the stress of surgery (213). Because of this common use of intraoperative opioids, the pupil is small and does not dilate following a nociceptive stimulus from surgical trauma (PRD). PRD can be used to indicate opioid effect during surgery (214; see also Chapter 12). With the combined effect of anesthetics and opioids, the pupil is small and has diminished light reflexes as measured in mm of constriction. And the LO reflex is absent because inhibition has been blocked. Even without the administration of opioids, general anesthesia will remove the inhibitory control of pupil size and block the LO response. As observed in Figure 10.16, there is essentially no prolonged dilation of the pupil in the anesthetized subject after the light is abruptly turned off.

Why is the pupil (in darkness) small during anesthesia in the absence of nociception? Consider the differences between the excitatory and inhibitory influences on the EW nucleus between the awake subject and the subject under general anesthesia. In both situations, the excitation by light is intact. However, inhibition from the arousal nuclei is lacking in the anesthetized subject, but is active in the awake subject (38, 39). So when the pupil is illuminated and then turned off, there is no underlying inhibition at the EW nucleus that would result in dilation of the pupil (Figure 10.16).

Another question then arises as to why the pupil during anesthesia should remain constricted when both the excitatory (light) and inhibitory (wakefulness) influences on that nucleus are absent. An in-depth study of sleep miosis was conducted on cats whose eyes were held open during sleep through a special lens that fits onto the corneal surface. To eliminate excitatory input to the EW nucleus, the optic nerves were severed to

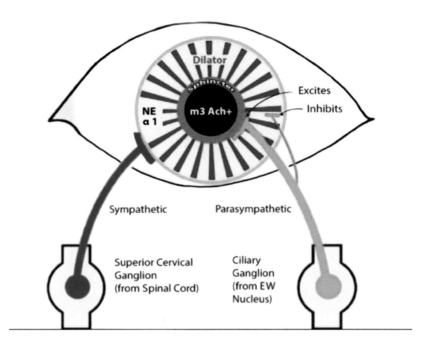

Figure 10.15 When the sphincter is activated to induce miosis, the sympathetic dilator is simultaneously inhibited (pathway shown in green). LO inhibits the EW nucleus and with a decrease in the firing rate of the ciliary ganglion, the dilator is released from inhibition and the pupil dilates. Drawing by Ping Hill, Research Intern, University of California, San Francisco.

produce blindness. As the authors demonstrated, the pupils were constricted in both synchronized and desynchronized sleep. There were small dilations that accompanied rapid eye movements and arousing stimulation that did not awaken the animals. This study therefore confirmed that the miosis observed during sleep or general anesthesia is not secondary to any special pharmacological property of the anesthetic agents, but is simply secondary to the loss of wakefulness and the removal of inhibitory influences on the EW nucleus (38, 39, 215, 216).

Several studies have concluded that the EW nucleus is spontaneously active in the absence of synaptic input. Lesions placed around the nucleus that sever afferent connections into the nucleus result in a rapid firing of the EW neurons and constriction of the pupil (217). This spontaneous activity also produces the miosis of sleep. LO does not dilate the pupil because there is no underlying inhibitory influence at the EW nucleus that (in the awake state) is brought about by the influence of the reticular formation nuclei.

Inhibition at the EW nucleus is blocked by opioids (134). Consequently, these drugs also block the LO reflex. In contrast to general anesthesia, it appears that opioids do not block the arousal centers directly, but they interfere with the inhibitory influence of these nuclei on the EW nucleus. Previous studies have demonstrated how opioids interfere with inhibitory transmission in the mesencephalon (218).

In this chapter, two measures, PUAL and the LO reflex, were described. Figure 10.17 illustrates the role of light and inhibition at the EW nucleus that produces PUAL and the

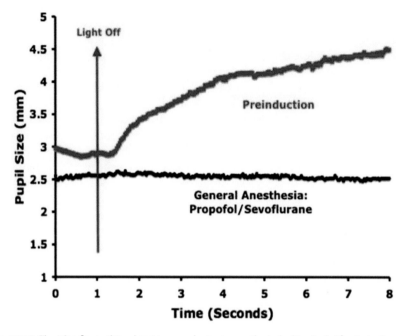

Figure 10.16 The LO reflex in this subject is normal prior to anesthesia (red tracing). After induction with propofol and sevoflurane, the LO reflex is nearly absent, only dilating a few tenths of a mm after the light is turned off. Pupillometry readings taken from a consenting patient.

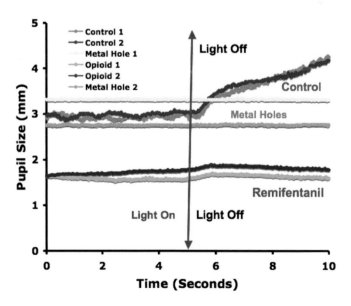

Figure 10.17 This image was produced by using the Neuroptics-3000 pupillometer to measure PUAL and the LO reflex in one 10-second scan. Explanation in the text. Pupillometer measurements were taken from a consenting volunteer subject.

LO reflex. Two measurements labeled control 1 and control 2 were taken prior to administration of remifentanil. From 0 to 5 seconds, light is directed into the measured eye and the pupil exhibits the typical waveform of PUAL. When the light is turned off at 5 seconds, the pupil dilates because of combined sympathetic activation and inhibition at the EW nucleus. The fluctuations are now absent because light is absent. The measurements labeled metal holes are included to show that a small amount of noise is inherent in the pupillometer.

Contrast the top measures with the two lower scans taken after remifentanil had been given in a dose to produce apnea. As before, light is directed into the measured eye, but inhibition at the EW nucleus has been blocked by the drug. Accordingly, there is no PUAL value with light on, and no sustained dilation at light off. The small 0.1 mm dilation represents the recovery phase of the light reflex that is not altered by the drug. Theoretically, this small dilation should be sustained at the diameter prior to the illumination of the pupil. Why the pupil tends to slowly constrict after the initial small dilation might be related to an after-image that persists after the light is turned off (219).

From these results with remifentanil infusions, it appears that sympathetic activation by itself cannot dilate the pupil at LO when the pupil is constricted by opioids. Presumably, the lack of sympathetic dilation is due to the block of the dilator muscle by the rapid firing rate of the EW nucleus (Figure 10.15). An examination of the combined effects of parasympathetic inhibition and sympathetic activation on the LO response was reported by Omary et al. (81). These authors noted that the early portion of the LO reflex was brought about by relaxation of the sphincter.

In summary, the LO reflex and PUAL require inhibitory activity at the EW nucleus. Sympathetic tone in the dilator muscle augments both parameters. Opioids depress and eventually block the LO reflex, PUAL, and PRD. Chapter 12 will provide a more complete discussion on the effect of opioids on the pupil.

Traumatic Brain Injury, Cardiac Arrest, Intensive Care

I tried to examine his pupils for signs of concussion. He foiled me by closing his eyes and tilting his head back.

(Diana Gabaldon, *Outlander, A Novel*)

The eyes were lifeless, and lusterless, and seemingly pupilless, and I shrank involuntarily from their glassy stare to the contemplation of the thin and shrunken lips. They parted, and in a smile of peculiar meaning, the teeth of the changed Berenice disclosed themselves slowly to my view. Would to God that I had never beheld them, or that, having done so, I had died!

(Edgar Allen Poe, *Berenice*)

Many neuro-intensive care units have incorporated portable pupillometers into their scheduled monitoring routines. Glasgow coma scales (GCS) (221) and Four Score evaluations (222) of brain-injured patients are commonly documented. Using the portable pupillometers, pupillary reactions and reflexes can readily be assessed by the nursing staff and entered into the electronic record. The pupillary reflexes add value to the GCS and the Four Score and can document more precise measures of pupillary reflexes compared to the traditional pen-light examination. The GCS and the Four Score scoring methods rely partially on motor responses. Because the pupillary reactions remain intact during loss of motor function, these scales can add value to the neurological assessment. This has an advantage when evaluating patients with possible cognitive–motor dissociation. A modified version of the GCS has been proposed that includes the quality of the pupillary light reflex (223).

The EW nucleus resides in the rostral portion of the midbrain, near the brain stem nuclei that control arousal. The cortico-spinal tracts that are essential for voluntary movement surround the periaqueductal gray. Important essential fiber tracts involved in motion, pain, sleep, blood pressure control, and breathing are in the nearby pons and medulla. The blood supply to this area arises from small penetrating arteries that arise from the vertebral-basilar artery and are frequently implicated in hypertensive-related infarcts and hemorrhage. Blunt trauma to the head can rupture these blood vessels and result in midbrain-related deficits. For these reasons, a trend of pupillary reflexes can be useful to clinicians who manage patients with vascular, hypoxic, or traumatic insults to the upper brain stem.

The recent literature on this topic is extensive. Many of the studies have concentrated on the prognostic value of various parameters of the pupillary light reflex (182, 224–248). This discussion will separate the pupillary findings associated with traumatic brain injury

(TBI) from those occurring after cardiac arrest. The pathophysiology of TBI is often related to intracranial lesions that result in compression of the brain stem, whereas the pupillary changes after cardiac arrest are related to lack of blood supply to the midbrain.

Lesions that arise from ischemic insults to the oculomotor nerve can result in "pupil sparing" syndromes that can produce strabismus and diplopia without mydriasis or pupillary areflexia. The oculomotor fibers that innervate four of the extraocular muscles are located within the core of the third nerve and can be damaged by diabetic and hypertensive infarcts. These lesions can spare the fibers that innervate the pupillary sphincter which are located on the surface of the nerve. The author will not discuss the literature relating to pupil sparing syndromes.

11.1 Traumatic Brain Injury

A common pupillary sign of brain trauma is a dilated and nonreactive pupil on the side of injury. This valuable sign was recognized in the late nineteenth century, and the description of this syndrome is a classic in the medical literature. Jonathan Hutchinson (1828–1913) was a British surgeon and ophthalmologist who described the phenomenon in 1878. His name is often associated with a pupil that is dilated and fixed to light and near vision (249). He frequently wrote manuscripts on the significance of pupillary examinations. As is typical of many contributors to our knowledge about the pupil, Hutchinson achieved notoriety in several fields of medicine, was knighted by the Queen, and wrote several textbooks and over 1,000 articles on various aspects of surgical technique.

Although there are several different syndromes and scenarios that alter the pupil after brain injury, one common scenario is thought to arise through the development of subdural hematomas that increase intracranial pressure and displace the brain into areas that compress the brain stem. Herniation of the brain from increased ICP can occur by different mechanisms. Uncal herniation typically compresses the third cranial nerve and produces pupillary dilation and loss of the light reflex. With the unilateral dilated and fixed pupil, we have one of the most valuable signs of cerebral edema or brain swelling, one that does not require any expensive equipment to recognize. A late ominous sign is bilateral fixed mydriasis. The pupil is usually dilated ipsilateral to the lesion, but that is not always true. Reports have documented pupillary dilation on the opposite side to the lesion (250). Case reports can provide insights into the relationship between increased intracranial pressure and pupillary reflex abnormalities (Figure 11.1; 233, 251).

Discrete lesions in the pons produce small pupils with a retained light reflex. Presumably, this pupillary syndrome comes about by interfering with the inhibitory influence of the lower pons on the EW nucleus. Finally, the cerebellar tonsils can be displaced onto the foramen magnum and compress the vital brain stem structures in the medulla. This is typically a catastrophic event that produces profound hypotension and depressed breathing with pupillary dilation from asphyxia. The five types of herniations of the brain and how they compress the third cranial nerve have been discussed in the neurology literature (12). Another cause of third nerve injury can develop from an aneurysm of the posterior communicating artery.

Several publications have reported on the use of portable infrared pupillometry in the management of TBI (226, 252–257). The initial paper that described the concept of NPi was a study of patients with increased intracranial pressure. The abbreviation NPi or

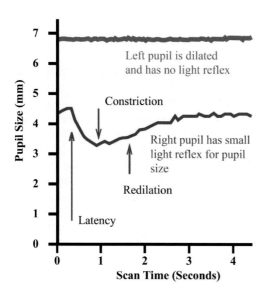

Left pupil is dilated
and has no light reflex

Constriction

Right pupil has small
light reflex for pupil
size

Redilation

Latency

Pupil Size (mm)

Scan Time (Seconds)

Figure 11.1 Pupillary scans taken from a patient with bilateral subdural hematomas; pupil is larger on the right. Permission to reproduce image granted from Wolters Kluwer Health, Inc. under License Number 501845673.

"Neurological Pupillary index" derives from studies on the light reflex with intracranial pathology (233). As a means to measure intracranial hypertension, pupillometers might provide the incentive to proceed to direct measurements of intracranial pressure that are continuous and more precise. Intracranial hypertension can be compartmentalized. If the pressures are not transmitted in a caudal direction, then direct ICP readings might be elevated without significant compression of the brain stem or alterations in third nerve function.

A recent summary of 60 cases of TBI with pupillary abnormalities reported that the most common cause was diffuse brain injury without lateralizing signs. Twenty-two percent of the patients with bilateral pupillary areflexia by the pen-light examination made a full recovery (255). More subtle changes in the size and reactivity of the pupil can be detected with infrared pupillometry. Confirmatory radiological evidence is always required before neurosurgical intervention is undertaken on a patient with head injury and a dilated, fixed pupil. Injuries to the brain frequently also include damage to the retina and optic nerve. Both the afferent and the efferent arms of the pupillary reflex can then be compromised after TBI. Recent reports have suggested that even mild degrees of TBI that do not progress to loss of consciousness can alter certain parameters of the pupillary light reflex (256, 257). Long-term pupillary abnormalities have been reported after TBI in patients who have clinically recovered, but these reports have not been confirmed (254).

11.2 Post Cardiac Arrest

And who art thou, boy? I see not my reflection in the vacant pupils of thy eyes. Oh God!!! That man should be a thing for immortal souls to sieve through! Who art thou, boy?

(Herman Melville, *Moby Dick*)

11.2.1 Prognostic Pupillary Measurements after Return of Spontaneous Circulation

Several studies have investigated the prognostic value of the pupillary light reflex after cardiac arrest, cardiopulmonary resuscitation (CPR), and extracorporeal membrane oxygenation (ECMO) (235–248; 258–276). Levy et al. (266) used a simple scoring system that included the presence or absence of the light reflex plus glucose concentrations, and found that the return of the light reflex predicted neurological recovery with a high degree of accuracy. Longstreth et al. (267) reached similar conclusions. Numerous factors contribute to pupillary dilation during cardiac arrest, including nociception, asphyxia, drugs, and severe brain stem hypoxia. As discussed previously, atropine even in standard doses does not produce fixed nonreactive pupils, although some dilation is observed (268). Recently, it has been shown that rapid cooling of the cardiac arrest patient can improve neurologic recovery. Because the light reflex is only minimally affected by mild hypothermia (17), it is possible that monitoring the light reflex of these paralyzed and mildly hypothermic post cardiac arrest patients could provide additional prognostic data during the hypothermic period. Profound hypothermia to below 30 degrees C depresses the light reflex and prevents prognostic value from pupillary light reflex measurements (145). A light reflex that progressively gains amplitude as the cardiac output is restored indicates a favorable prognosis, but if the reflex is small and does not change within the first few hours, then the patient very often will have an unfavorable prognosis. Absent pupillary light reflexes 72 hours after return of spontaneous circulation (ROSC) predicts a poor prognosis with nearly 100 percent certainty (268, 269), but abnormal pupillary syndromes should always be considered.

A pupillometric test that predicts awakening after cardiac arrest with a high sensitivity and a high specificity has not been reported (240, 270, 271). Kondziella has recently reviewed this literature (273). Absent pupillary light reflexes 72 hours after cardiac arrest indicates a high specificity for a poor outcome, but sensitivity is only 30 percent (273). An NPi below 2 has 100 percent specificity for determining a poor outcome with only 32 percent specificity. A combination of neurological tests and various times after ROSC can be predictive of neurological function after 3 months. Prognosis following ROSC is typically determined by combining the clinical examination with physiological measurements and serum biomarkers (274). Here, the value of infrared pupillometry seems obvious. A depressed light reflex can sometimes be detected with the pupillometer, but is not appreciated by the standard pen-light examination. Even a small light reflex is indicative of intact brain stem function and might alter the prognosis.

The traditional pen-light examination of the pupils during and after resuscitation is not as predictive for a good outcome as measurements taken with an infrared pupillometer (237). Additionally, a parameter of the light reflex that is independent of the pupil size, such as the NPi, is more useful than the extent of the reflex in mm. As with other measures of neurological function, a single measurement is not as valuable as the trend of values over time.

The neocortex is more vulnerable to anoxic insults than the midbrain. A patient might therefore have return of midbrain reflexes, including the pupillary light reflex, but have extensive damage to the neocortex. These patients often have extensive neurological deficits after return of the light reflex. The measurement of a midbrain reflex does not precisely indicate the status of the oxygenation of neocortical structures. For several reasons, using the PLR alone for prognosis is not recommended. The 2020 American Heart Association guidelines do mention the value of infrared pupillometry 72 hours after ROSC as an additional measure to predict prognosis (270).

The pupillary reactions after cardiac arrest are useful to consider, but a study of hundreds of cases of cardiac arrest cannot help the clinician to precisely predict the future course of any one individual case. Physicians deal with a single patient and the family of that patient. A battery of tests that include the pupillary measurements together with information from serum biomarkers and EEG recordings can provide a range of possible outcomes, and this information can be presented to family for discussion (274–276).

11.2.2 Prognostic Value of Pupillary Measurements During Cardiopulmonary Resuscitation

Pupil size and pupillary reaction to light during CPR have been measured in animals. Binnion and McFarland noted in dogs that 30 percent of normal cardiac output is sufficient to constrict the dilated pupil during cardiac arrest (277). Sobotka and Gebert measured the pupil after induced cardiac arrest in dogs. They observed maximum pupillary dilation 5 minutes after cessation of the circulation, and restoration of cardiac output produced pupillary constriction (278). Zhao et al. examined the predictive value of pupillary light reflexes during induced cardiac arrest and cardiopulmonary resuscitation in pigs. Intact light reflexes and pupillary constriction predicted ROSC and good neurological outcomes, whereas absent light reflexes predicted poor outcomes. If pupillary reflexes were absent for over 6 minutes during CPR, then the outcomes were consistently poor (123).

Pupillary measurements have been taken in humans during cardiopulmonary resuscitation. Steen-Hansen et al. measured the pupil during 244 cases of resuscitation during cardiac arrest and described the pupillary changes by using a pen light. With 13.5 percent of these cases, a light reflex was present; 31 percent were uncertain; and, with the remainder, the light reflex was thought to be absent. Patients in whom the light reflex was present had a more favorable outcome compared to those with no reflex during CPR (279). More recently, Kim et al. measured the light reflex during CPR in out-of-hospital cardiac arrest cases and correlated the NPi values during resuscitation to survival with favorable neurological outcomes. These results suggested that an NPi of higher than 2 indicated an early favorable outcome of the out-of-hospital cardiac arrest cases (280). These citations refer to research studies only. The most recent guidelines by the American Heart Association regarding cardiopulmonary resuscitation do not mention pupillometry during CPR (281).

To evaluate the quality of the light reflex with a portable instrument during CPR requires an experienced operator and one that has a full understanding of CPR techniques. Delaying chest compressions to take light reflex measurements is unacceptable. The pupillary measurements must be taken within less than 6 seconds, requiring skill with the instrument and an understanding of potential risks to the cornea from improper technique. Brief pauses occur during ACLS for evaluation of the EKG rhythm, for airway manipulation, and for auscultation of the chest (Figure 11.2). These are appropriate intervals to evaluate the pupil. The return of the light reflex during CPR and before ROSC has not been studied with many patients, but preliminary case reports suggest that if the reflex returns during CPR, this would predict a favorable outcome (Figures 11.3 and 11.4; 282).

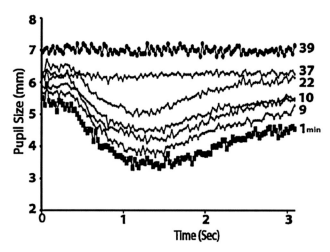

Figure 11.2 It is possible to measure the pupillary light reflex during cardiopulmonary resuscitation. Measurements can be taken briefly when chest compressions are paused to examine the electrocardiogram and examine the pulse. The patient from whom these scans were taken had a massive pulmonary embolus and could not be resuscitated. The anesthesiologist managed the airway and measured the pupil when the team was not compressing the chest. Note the progressive dilation of the pupil and the loss of the light reflex as neuronal death within the EW nucleus progresses. The code was called after 40 minutes of resuscitation. Permission to reproduce image obtained from Elsevier under License Number 5593310287599.

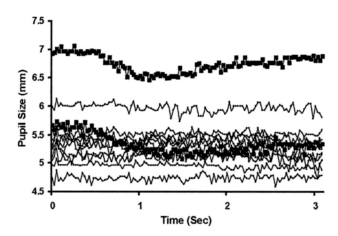

Figure 11.3 This patient was resuscitated with chest compressions for 39 minutes before ROSC was established. The thin black lines were taken during assessment of the EKG and showed absent light reflexes. Three minutes after ROSC, the pupillary reflexes returned and are shown by the bold black pupillary scans. By inserting these reflex parameters into the graph illustrated in Figure 8.4, it is noted that these reflexes are markedly depressed. The patient died on the second post arrest day without regaining consciousness. Permission to reproduce image obtained from Elsevier under License Number 5593310287599.

Continued improvement in the quality of the light reflex might indicate that the chest compressions are perfusing the midbrain with oxygenated blood, whereas progressive loss of the light reflex would suggest a failed resuscitation (Figure 11.2). After ROSC,

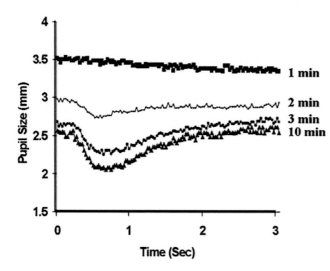

Figure 11.4 If during CPR a normal light reflex returns quickly, then the patient typically recovers without neurological deficits. By 2 minutes after chest compressions, the light reflex had returned. This patient had no residual neurological deficit. Permission to reproduce image obtained from Elsevier under License Number 5593310287599.

it is valuable to record the time to the return of the light reflex into the normal range. Trending the return of the light reflex is more useful than an isolated measure.

An absent pupillary light reflex should never be used to discontinue resuscitation efforts (279). This would be a flaw in management. The extent of the PLR in patients prior to cardiac arrest is unknown. There are rare cases of awake patients having no PLR, but who are otherwise neurologically intact. Therefore, a thorough history of each patient is essential. Patients that are blind from glaucoma, extensive macular degeneration, or advanced diabetic retinopathy would have depressed light reflexes or possibly no light reflex. Also, there are patients with tonic reflexes. See Bremner and Smith for a discussion of the causes of these reflexes (283). They are characterized by low amplitudes and low constriction velocities. Of course, these patients represent a very small percentage of the population, but the physician must be aware of these confounding syndromes. The PLR is useful, but should not be used alone to guide therapy during and after resuscitation.

Pupils are typically at midposition after death (284, 285). The large pupil size at the moment of death might be secondary to a surge of norepinephrine release. The pupil dilates following cross-clamping of the aorta during organ retrieval from brain-dead patients. Clearly, this is a result of asphyxia. Because topical dapiprazole, an alpha 1 adrenergic antagonist, blocks this dilation, it appears to be brought about by a sympathetic mechanism (125). This latter explanation is consistent with the observations of Loewenfeld, who observed sympathetically mediated dilation immediately following the death of experimental animals (39).

11.3 Cognitive–Motor Dissociation

In neuro-intensive care units, there are a small group of patients who appear to be unaware, but because of depressed motor function are minimally conscious. Various forms of cognitive–motor dissociation can prevent patients from initiating a motor response to verbal instructions. One example is the locked in syndrome. It has become apparent that nearly 15 percent of comatose patients have a syndrome of cognitive–motor dissociation that prevents the healthcare worker from determining the state of consciousness. These patients appear to be unconscious, but might be totally awake. The issue is sometimes studied with functional MRI or EEG patterns following requests for a mental exercise. These methods are time-consuming and expensive, so other simple tests are under consideration. Patients who are classified as either in a vegetative or minimally conscious state sometimes pass in and out of consciousness. Highly technical and time-consuming methods to ascertain if a subject is aware of their environment capture only one point in time and might not detect the waxing and waning of consciousness (286, 287).

An intact pupillary light reflex does not imply that a patient is awake, because drug-induced coma with propofol and opioids has minimal effects on the PLR (135). But there is a need for easy recognition of the awake state in patients who lack motor function. There might be a role for portable infrared pupillometry to detect the presence of cognitive–motor dissociation. Vassilieva et al. have measured task-evoked dilations in brain-injured patients with minimal levels of consciousness. A multiplication problem was presented to these patients and pupil sizes were measured between 15 and 30 seconds with the Neuroptics PLR-3000. They observed a slow dilation that occurred after the multiplication problem was presented (287). These types of studies might be used in neuro-intensive care units to detect residual consciousness in patients with cognitive–motor dissociation. The classical example is a patient who has a brain injury and is paralyzed with neuromuscular blocking agents to prevent coughing or straining during mechanical ventilation. Of course, there are EEG and fMRI techniques to answer these questions. However, pupillometry is easy to perform and not time-consuming or expensive.

A recently published article describes the use of brimonidine eye drops to evaluate whether subjects are conscious or not conscious. As noted previously, the dilator muscle of the iris is not active during unconscious states (39, 99). Consequently, blocking the sympathetic innervation of the iris dilator would not constrict the pupil if patients are unconscious, but would do so in awake subjects. Jakobsen et al. studied 15 normal awake volunteers and 15 patients who were determined to be unconscious by electroencephalography, clinical evaluation, and fMRI criteria. The pupils constricted after brimonidine topical eye drops in awake volunteers, but failed to constrict in unconscious patients (288). This was a preliminary study that will require confirmation. It does suggest a method to assess residual awareness that does not rely on cumbersome monitoring devices such as fMRI. As discussed in Chapter 8, general anesthesia has unusual effects on the waveform of the light reflex, possibly related to the loss of sympathetic tone in the dilator muscle. However, a complete study of the LO reflex in unconscious patients who lack sympathetic tone has not been conducted. Future studies on this topic will test the hypothesis that a patient with PUAL values in the range of normal with a sustained LO reflex confirms a state of wakefulness.

Chapter 12

Opioid Effect and Acute Pain

For many years he continued to be a slave to the drug, an object of mingled horror and pity to his friends and relatives. I can see him now, with yellow, pasty face, drooping lids, and pin-point pupils, all huddled in a chair, the wreck and ruin of a noble man.

(Sir Arthur Conan Doyle, *The Adventures of Sherlock Holmes: Adventure VI. The Man with the Twisted Lip*)

12.1 History of Opioid Miosis

The ability of opioids to constrict the pupil is an old observation. Almost 300 years ago, Fontana described how these drugs constrict the pupil in his classic paper on the movements of the iris (31). It is a confusing topic because experimental animals have unusual pupillary effects after opioid administration (187). The effects of anesthetics, sedatives, and opioids on pupil size depend on the species under study (289). For the clinician, it is not important to know that the cat pupil dilates after morphine or that in rabbits and mice opioids induce pupillary fluctuations, sometimes in synchrony with the EEG (186, 187). The human pupil constricts to small diameters after opioids and during general anesthesia. These small diameters are observed both in darkness and in light. Several manuscripts confirm this observation (18, 55).

The miosis after opioid use is not precisely "pinpoint" as is often described in the popular literature. Even with a toxic overdose of opioids, the pupil rarely constricts to diameters below 2 mm. The mean diameter during toxic overdose is 2.2 ± 0.26 (140) to 2.5 ± 0.20 mm (290). Stimulation with bright light will constrict the pupil another 0.1 to 0.2 mm after opioid overdose becomes apparent (see Figure 12.3). The "pinpoint" pupil has also been reported to occur after localized lesions in the pons. Accurate measurements of the diameter with pontine lesions have never been described (12). In addition, there are no studies that have asked whether the light reflexes in these cases are within normal limits as described in Chapter 8. The term "pinpoint" should probably be retired from the vocabulary of medicine because it is not a defined measure. The pupil can constrict to diameters below 1 mm following topical application of pilocarpine, but what diameter is meant by the term "pinpoint" has never been explained (39, 291).

Nevertheless, with attention to detail, it is apparent that the human pupil is exquisitely sensitive to the miotic effect of opioids. But if the pupil is already constricted in the presence of bright light, additional opioid in that setting would have almost no effect on the diameter of the pupil (292, 293). It is also useful to consider concurrent medications that have anticholinergic properties (294), thus preventing opioid-induced constriction of the pupil.

Opioids have multiple effects on the human body. They depress respiration (295), promote nausea, ablate pain, constrict the pupil, reduce peristalsis, and induce drowsiness. Each of these effects has different dose response characteristics and duration of action. The ability of opioids to constrict the dark-adapted pupil has been used as a pharmacodynamic measure to assess the central nervous system effects of opioids (296–301).

12.2 Mechanism of Opioid Effect on the Pupil

Why do opioids constrict the pupil? Several years ago, it was noted that topical morphine constricted the pupil. The conjecture was that these drugs constricted the pupil by acting on the iris musculature and that topical naloxone would dilate the pupil of morphine addicts (302). It was thought, therefore, that the action to constrict the pupil was an ocular phenomenon that was not related to a central effect of the drug.

The idea that these drugs act on the iris was discredited by the observation that large doses of intravenous opioids did not constrict the pupils of brain-dead patients (303). Furthermore, it was shown that transection of the oculomotor nerve abolished the effect of opioids on the pupil (14). Patients with Horner's syndrome have small pupils, but they constrict further after the administration of opioids (47). All of this information lends support to the theory that an increased firing rate of the EW neurons is responsible for constriction of the pupil after these drugs.

An appreciation of how opioids constrict the pupil is crucial if the physicism wants to benefit from infrared pupillometry as a measure of opioid effect. Historically, it has been taught that opioids increased the activity of the EW neurons. Lee and Wang, for example, recorded the efferent activity of the EW neurons in dogs anesthetized with nitrous oxide and oxygen. They observed that the administration of morphine produced a rapid firing rate in these neurons that was concomitant with pupillary constriction. Cervical sympathectomy did not interfere with the miotic response. Thus, a sympathetic block was not sufficient to observe the pupillary constriction. The drug also constricted the pupil in dogs whose cerebral hemispheres had been removed. Levallorphan, an opioid antagonist, reversed all of the effects on the pupil by morphine. These authors concluded that morphine produced an excitatory action on the EW nucleus (14).

It is important to note that these dogs were paralyzed and only partially anesthetized with nitrous oxide. Morphine in this case might have added to the sedative effect of nitrous oxide and thus induced a more sleep-like state with accompanying miosis of sleep. It is well known, however, that opioids constrict the pupil irrespective of inducing sleep.

A review article in 1983 by Duggan and North on the electrophysiology of opioid effects described the depressant effect that these agents have as they interact with opioid receptors in the brain (304). This article concluded that any excitatory effect of these agents was brought about by a process of disinhibition . . . for example, inhibition of an inhibitory pathway. Opioids hyperpolarize membranes by activation of a potassium conductance and depress calcium-induced release of neurotransmitters (218, 304).

It had been known since the classic studies of Loewenfeld (13) that the dilation of the pupil that occurred during general anesthesia was brought about by inhibition of the EW

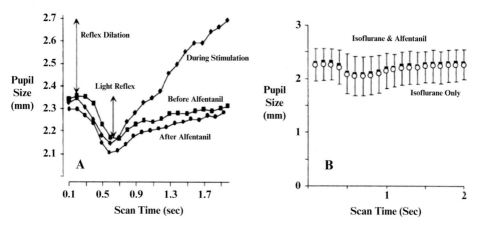

Figure 12.1 A bolus of alfentanil during anesthesia does not alter the light reflex (A and B). A noxious stimulus will dilate the pupil in the absence of opioids (A). Permission to reproduce image was obtained from Wolters Kluwer Health, Inc., under License Number 5593160241753.

nucleus. This was confirmed in human studies in 1993 through the observation that PRD was the same size in both pupils even when the dilator muscles of one eye had been blocked by alpha 1 adrenergic blockade (99). It was apparent then that PRD during anesthesia is an inhibitory process at the EW nucleus and that opioids block this inhibition (134), thereby blocking PRD during anesthesia. Also, during general anesthesia in the absence of nociception, opioids do not constrict the pupil. And they do not increase or decrease the amplitude of the light reflex (Figure 12.1). Additional light directed into the pupil can constrict the pupil under the same conditions (215). These studies suggest that any alteration in PLR amplitude by the opioids is dependent on limiting the mechanical range of the pupil (305). Thus, the mechanism by which opioids constrict the pupil is not brought about by excitation of the EW nucleus, but rather by blocking the inhibitory influences that impinge on the nucleus during the awake state.

Figure 9.4 illustrates this effect of opioids in blocking inhibitory influences on the EW nucleus. This property of opioids can be used as a simple diagnostic test. Seventy-five micrograms of intravenous fentanyl should constrict the dark diameter of the pupil to below 3 mm except in certain clinical settings. These exceptions include the unusual pupillary syndromes (Chapter 5), third nerve compression, or extreme asphyxia. One other diagnosis would be opioid tolerance. The miotic effects of opioids exhibit tolerance just like the respiratory depressant effects (306). Blindness would not alter the ability of opioids to constrict the pupil.

12.3 Importance of Pupillometry to Management of Opioid Therapy

Although opioids for pain management are used less frequently than they were 20 years ago, they remain essential drugs for severe pain. Opioid-related deaths still occur in the hospital and at home under the direct supervision of physicians (307). Patients who report postoperative pain are typically offered non-opioid analgesics such as nerve blocks, gabapentin, acetaminophen, and NSAIDs as the first line of therapy. Failing those therapies, opioids are used and, even though adjunctive therapies are improving, many patients still require opioids in the immediate postoperative period. It is not a benign therapy in patients who receive these drugs through multiple sources, which in some patients might include epidural, intravenous, and oral routes of administration. Compounding the problem for the clinician is the wide variability in the response to opioid-induced respiratory depression from the same dose of the drug (308).

Because of the variability in response, a measure of opioid effect can be useful. Opioid titration is not always as simple as using intermittent measurements of respiratory rate. Oximeters and end-tidal CO_2 monitors can be dislodged or improperly adjusted. One difficult management case, for example, is the patient with an opioid intrathecal pump that is discontinued because of malfunction or infection. These patients are at risk for withdrawal if intravenous or oral opioid replacements are mismanaged. For these reasons, pupillometry can add to the clinical management of patients on opioid therapy.

Opioids can be given orally, intravenously, transdermally, and intramuscularly. One often overlooked route of delivery is via neuraxial administration. Many patients on the acute pain service have epidural catheters through which a mixture of local anesthetics and opioids is administered to treat acute postoperative pain. The original idea of using epidural and spinal opioids was to directly place the opioid agonist onto the opioid receptors in the dorsal horn and thereby decrease the transmission from the primary afferent to the secondary neuron in the nociceptive pathway. The first reports of spinal opioids were published in 1979, but within a few years it became apparent that spinal opioids have the potential for producing systemic effects that can be life-threatening (Case Report 12.1). Morphine is distributed preferentially in the CSF and can depress the respiratory center through migration within the neuroaxis. Other more fat-soluble opioids like fentanyl can be absorbed into the circulation and produce respiratory depression, like a slow intravenous infusion. With the current emphasis on postoperative opioid-sparing methods, the use of serial measures of pupillary unrest in ambient light (PUAL) can be useful. A daily objective measure of opioid effect will confirm that the goal of opioid sparing has been successful.

One study examined the depression of PRD brought about by epidural fentanyl administered in the T10–T11 interspace. The volunteers were mechanically ventilated and under general anesthesia. Epidural fentanyl was administrated as a bolus injection into the T10 interspace and produced reduction of PRD from stimulation of electrodes placed on the C5 dermatome. The depression from the C5 stimulation site was nearly as profound as that observed from stimulating the L4 dermatome. The PRD depression from 1 mcg/kg of epidural fentanyl was maximal at 45 minutes, indicating a slow absorption from the epidural site compared to the same dose administered intravenously, the effect of which peaked at 6 minutes (173).

12.4 Pupillary Measures of Opioid Effect

The relationship between respiratory depression and portable infrared pupillary measurements has been studied and the most sensitive parameters that indicate opioid effect have been documented. During general anesthesia, the value of depression of pupillary reflex dilation has been documented as a measure of opioid effect. This topic has already been discussed in Chapter 9.

Case Report 12.1

A patient was observed on the first postoperative day following a Whipple procedure for bile duct carcinoma. A thoracic epidural infusion of ropivacaine and dilaudid 10 mcg/cc was running at 6 cc/hr. Her pain scores were 2–3/10 and she had no complaints. On postoperative day 2, she was vomiting and mildly sedated, which she attributed to lack of sleep. The infusion rate and epidural solution were the same, but PUAL was now depressed to about half of the value registered on postoperative day 1. With the idea that this depression of PUAL might represent the effect of dilaudid, the decision was made to remove the opioid from the epidural mixture. On postoperative day 3, the vomiting had subsided, and she was more alert. Pain was still controlled to the patient's satisfaction with epidural local anesthetic alone, and PUAL values were in the range of normal for her age.

In awake subjects, there are several measures derived from the pupil that can be used to estimate opioid effect. Aissou et al. observed that pressure on the abdomen after abdominal surgery will produce pupillary dilation, with the extent of the dilation correlating to the proper dose of opioid required to control pain for that subject (163). Another method is to measure the amount of current required to dilate the pupil 13 percent above baseline. This method has been discussed in Chapter 6 as a feature of the Algiscan pupillometer in PPI mode. The small currents are normally well tolerated by patients. Overall, however, adding a noxious stimulus in the awake patient is counterintuitive, and more benign measures of opioid effect in the awake patient have been studied.

In theory, a measurement of pupil size might be a useful clinical observation to follow the central effects of opioids. Dark-adapted pupil size might be used as a measure of opioid effect, but it is cumbersome to use in the clinical setting. There are other reasons why pupil size is not a good clinical test for opioid use in the general population. First, there are many patients who have small pupils even before the administration of opioids. Figure 12.2 illustrates five patients with small pupils who were not on opioids, not diabetic, and not over the age of 60. Some patients are born with small pupils. Other patients might have senile miosis or diabetes, or be taking topical medications. The miotic pupil is not a specific sign for opioid use. As discussed in the following paragraphs, more precise measures of opioid effect can be obtained by measuring PUAL or the LO reflex.

The problem with observing the pupil size for opioid effect with a pen light is the amount of ambient light that is required to see the pupil. Subjects with a very dark iris present a difficulty for the examiner because even to see the pupil, a light must be directed into the pupil prior to the estimation of the pupil size. If a high-intensity light is required just to see the pupil, then the pupil might be small even prior to opioid administrations. A consistent technique that is used by everyone taking pupillary measurements is essential (309). Portable infrared pupillometry removes the ambient light consideration because measurements with this technique can be made in total darkness. But it does not solve the issues surrounding the patients who have small pupils prior to opioid therapy. Even with doses of opioids that produce apnea, the pupil will not constrict much below a diameter of 2 mm. This means that if the pupil was 2.5 mm prior to opioid administration, it will constrict to its limiting diameter with only a small dose of opioid, and further opioid therapy will not reflect the increasing central effect of the drug. As mentioned

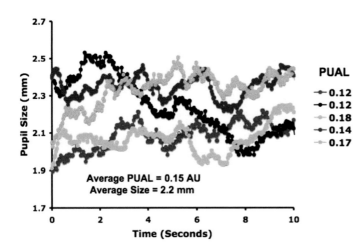

Figure 12.2 Several cases in the author's database exhibited small miotic pupils with no evidence of opioid effect. These patients had small pupils, but had normal values of PUAL. Pupillometer measurements from the author's files, taken from consenting patients.

previously in this chapter, many pharmacodynamic studies of opioid effect have been conducted on dark-adapted subjects. While this is a scientifically rigorous method to perform these studies, it is an impractical solution to use in the clinical setting.

There are also limitations to the use of the pupillary light reflex as a measure of opioid effect. Opioids constrict the pupil and thereby restrict the mechanical range that the pupil can move in response to the light stimulus. In most patients, pupil size begins to limit the light reflex amplitude at about 3 mm. The evidence seems clear, then, that constriction amplitude and pupil size will show a decrease in value as the pupil constricts following opioid therapy, but this decrease in both parameters simply reflects the mechanical limitation of the iris movement.

One method of overcoming this problem is that instead of using light reflex amplitude, it might be more accurate to use "percent constriction." But this idea is also fallacious. Percent constriction does decrease following opioid therapy, but the reflex is still present when severe respiratory depression occurs (Figure 12.3). As a remifentanil infusion produces an increasing opioid central effect, the percent reflex decreased from 45 to 15 percent as shown in Figure 12.3. This occurs because of the change in pupil size. This lack of effect by opioids on the light reflex is confirmed by the observation that there is no alteration of the NPi by administration of toxic doses of remifentanil (Figure 12.4). Clearly, other measures retrieved from the pupillometer might be more useful in detecting opioid effect in the awake patient. The value of PUAL becomes apparent because it is suppressed to zero as toxic levels of remifentanil develop (Figure 12.5; 310).

Chapter 10 discussed the importance of inhibitory influences on the EW nucleus to the generation of PUAL. These inhibitory influences are blocked progressively by opioids and thus provide a useful clinical measure of opioid effect in awake subjects. The mechanism by which opioids decrease inhibition at the EW nucleus is unknown. This depression might possibly be related to the known depressant effect that opioids have on inhibitory transmission in the pons (218, 311). Opioids are also known to depress activity in the locus coeruleus, which has been implicated as a source of inhibition of the EW nucleus (312).

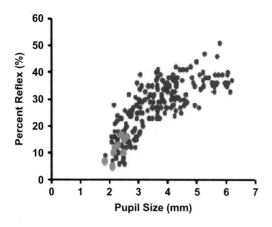

Figure 12.3 The percent reflex decreases as opioids diminish the size of the pupil. But percent reflex remains positive as subjects become apneic from opioid overdose. Subjects with apnea are shown with blue markers. Permission to reproduce image granted by Elsevier under the terms of the Creative Commons CC BY License, which permits unrestricted reproduction in any medium.

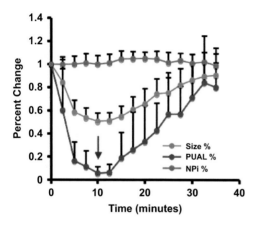

Figure 12.4 Administration of a toxic dose of remifentanil decreases PUAL to values near to zero. NPi is unchanged, and the size of the pupil decrease is limited by the mechanical constraints of the iris muscle and stroma. Permission to reproduce image granted by Elsevier under the terms of the Creative Commons CC BY License, which permits unrestricted reproduction in any medium.

Figures 12.4 and 12.5 show that PUAL is suppressed to zero as severe respiratory depression develops. Similarly, the LO reflex depends on inhibitory activity at the EW nucleus. Profound respiratory depression from remifentanil infusions will also ablate the LO reflex (Figure 12.6).

The 16-second measurement of pupil size shown in Figure 12.7 illustrates that opioids block inhibition at the EW nucleus, but leave the light reflex intact. The top (red) measurement was taken prior to the administration of a toxic infusion of remifentanil. Note the weak dilation in the first 3 seconds as the pupillometer was positioned over the measured eye and the opposite eye occluded from light by the operator's hand. After 3 seconds, a 3-second light stimulus of 1,000 lux was presented and a normal amplitude constriction of the pupil follows. Six seconds after the start of the measurement, the light was turned off and a 10-second "light off" dilation of 2.5 mm is observed. This measurement therefore shows that excitation by light on and inhibition by light off are both intact. The LO response is augmented by intact sympathetic tone in the dilator muscle.

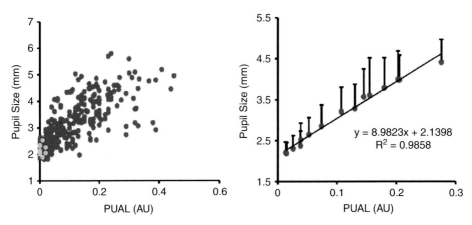

Figure 12.5 The relationship between pupil size and PUAL is distinctly different from that observed from percent constriction or constriction velocity. Note the values in blue that represent the PUAL values at the time of severe respiratory depression. PUAL values decrease to zero as respiratory depression develops after remifentanil infusions. Permission to reproduce image granted by Elsevier under the terms of the Creative Commons CC BY License, which permits unrestricted reproduction in any medium.

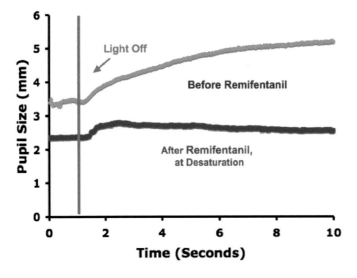

Figure 12.6 Before remifentanil, the LO reflex was robust and the dilation was not complete after 9 seconds. After remifentanil at the time of oxyhemoglobin desaturation, the early dilation shows the light reflex recovery, but the end pupil size does not show continued dilation that would represent the process of dark adaption. Unpublished pupillometry measurements taken from a consenting volunteer.

Contrast that with the measurement taken after remifentanil was administered to produce apnea (bottom [blue] tracing). The subject was awake and oxyhemoglobin saturation was falling below 90 percent. Nasal oxygen was started, and the subject was prompted to breathe. This measurement shows that excitation by light is intact, but there is no "light off" reflex, indicating the lack of inhibitory tone at the EW nucleus. The light reflex amplitude is normal for that size pupil (see Figure 8.4). Both the pre-drug and the post-drug measurements demonstrate that the "light off" response is a recovery from the "light on" reflex. But the pre-drug measurement shows continued pupillary dilation, whereas the post-drug measurement shows a gradual constriction.

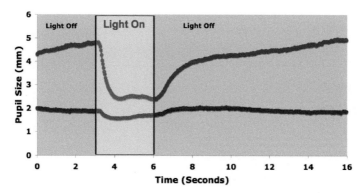

Figure 12.7 This measurement was taken from an unpublished volunteer study of 10 subjects who consented to receive high-dose remifentanil infusions (147). This subject was a 28-year-old male in good health. The red tracing is prior to the drug and the blue tracing is after the administration of remifentanil. Further explanation of the study is presented in the text.

These two previous illustrations show that the dilator muscle is not activated by "light off" during opioid toxicity because it is inhibited by the highly active pupilloconstrictor nerve. It is apparent from these observations that opioids do not eliminate inhibition by blocking wakefulness, but they do interfere with the process whereby wakefulness inhibits the nucleus. On the other hand, the elimination of the LO reflex during anesthesia and discussed in Chapter 10 presumably results from absence of the awake state.

12.5 Interaction Effects on Opioid-Induced Respiratory Depression, PUAL, and LO

Respiratory depression following opioid therapy is known to be antagonized by inter-action with the subject and by pain (313). Over 80 years ago, for example, Lundy observed that patients with kidney stones who were treated with opioids would some-times become apneic when the stone was passed (314). Patients with somnolence and respiratory depression from opioids can be aroused by bodily movement and interaction with friends and colleagues. A common scenario is when a caregiver asks questions and engages in a conversation with a patient after the administration of opioids. The caregiver then leaves the room only to be summoned by an alarm that the patient has low oxyhemoglobin saturation. Without continual interaction with the patient, opioids will influence the respiratory pattern and patients can become apneic. A pupillary measure of opioid effect that would not be altered by pain or by patient interaction would be a useful addition to the clinical use of these drugs. Such a measure would allow the clinician to predict opioid effect after the pain or interaction is absent.

McKay et al. studied the effect of engaging volunteers with conversation during remifentanil infusions on pupillary measurements (315). The same volunteer was studied twice, first with conversational interaction, and then a second infusion when the volun-teer was not disturbed. The non-interactive session was interrupted by periods of apnea and oxyhemoglobin desaturation, whereas the interactive group was less affected by the same infusion scheme (Figure 12.8). The changes in PUAL were the same during both

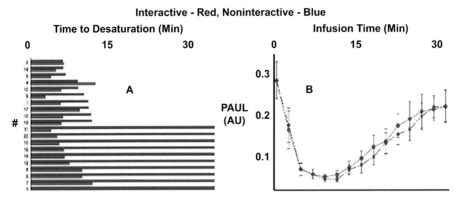

Figure 12.8 A: Fewer volunteers who were engaged in conversation (red lines) exhibited oxyhemoglobin desaturation. In addition, the time to oxyhemoglobin desaturation was longer with conversational engagement compared to the same dose of the drug given without conversational engagement (blue lines). Y axis is volunteer number, x axis is time in minutes. B: The changes in PUAL were the same with both experimental conditions. Permission to reproduce this figure was obtained from Springer under a Creative Commons Attribution 4.0 International License, which permits reproduction in any medium.

trials, indicating that PUAL is a measure of opioid effect in the presence of interaction with caregivers.

Very low values of PUAL can alert the caregiver that opioid effect is at a high level even when pain and other interactions with the patient might suggest otherwise. When interaction is removed, then dangerous respiratory depression can occur (315, 316). Another scenario is the patient who still has high pain scores after repeated doses of opioids. Surgical and nursing colleagues might then request the acute pain service to insert an epidural or a peripheral nerve block to decrease pain scores. When this is done, there is danger that respiratory depression might follow the block, particularly if an intense opioid effect is observed with pupillometry prior to the local anesthetic block. As previously discussed, pain antagonizes the respiratory depressant effect of opioids (316), and when the pain is removed, the full effect of opioid respiratory depression can become apparent. Escalation of opioid therapy for pain when there is already evidence of strong opioid effect can be futile (317) and lead to profound respiratory depression if regional blocks are added (compare Case Reports 12.2 and 12.3).

In experimental animals, it is possible to insert electrodes directly into the brain and then record the neuronal activity in the pupillary control system (54, 55, 311, 318). This is impossible in humans for obvious reasons, and because the pupils of humans respond differently to opioids compared to experimental animals, it is necessary to make inferences based on experimental procedures that can be performed on humans. Figure 12.9 illustrates the effect of pain and interaction on respiratory drive and the lack of effect on PUAL.

Cases like this suggest that patients who are opioid-tolerant and on opioids can have PUAL values within the range of normal and this reflects their tolerance to the effects of these drugs. The value of PUAL measurements at this juncture is to differentiate between drug-seeking behavior and actual effective opioid therapy. Effective opioid therapy will reduce PUAL, but if this does not occur, then pain relief will usually not be apparent (317).

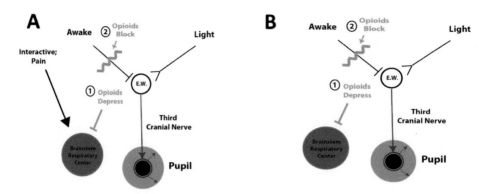

Figure 12.9 A: In the awake subject, stimulation of the respiratory center by pain or interaction with a caregiver will overcome the respiratory depressant effect of opioids (1). These factors will not change the depressant effect of opioids on PUAL (2). B: But when pain or interaction are not present, the full depressant effect of opioids on the respiratory center will become apparent and severe hypoventilation might develop. PUAL is not affected by pain or caregiver interaction. Image created by the author.

Case Report 12.2

The patient was a middle-aged opioid-tolerant female with a flare of endometriosis. Prior to hospital admission, she was taking methadone and dilaudid prn. 24-hour morphine equivalent was 200 mg. Other in-hospital non-opioid therapies, which included Neurontin, ketamine, PCA, amitriptyline, NSAIDs, and IV Tylenol, were ineffective. Clearly, this patient presented a therapeutic challenge that could be managed with several different methods. The acute pain service considered that her pain was severe enough to require frequent intermittent injections of dilaudid. The acute pain service was in continuous attendance while these injections were administered every 5 minutes. Prior to drug therapy, pupil size was 4.5 mm and PUAL was within the range of normal, even though she was taking the 24-hour equivalent of 200 mg of morphine daily. As the intravenous drug began to diminish her pain after 40 mg of dilaudid, the size of the pupil decreased only 0.5 mm, or 5 percent, whereas PUAL changed from 0.60 to 0.12, a decrease of 80 percent.

Of the common measures that are retrieved from portable pupillometers, the PUAL is most valuable because it approaches a value of zero at the level of opioid toxicity. The percent light reflex and constriction velocity remain positive even as total apnea appears. The zero value of PUAL after opioid therapy is simply a measure of the extent of profound opioid effect and is associated with marked respiratory depression. On the other hand, natural sleep and general anesthesia also depress PUAL to zero, but do not produce respiratory arrest. The low value of PUAL after opioid therapy simply implies that opioid effect is substantial, and caution is advised if interactive engagements (including pain) are removed.

12.6 Pain and PUAL Values

Opioids constrict and acute intense pain dilates the pupil. The question then arises as to what size the pupil becomes when pain is severe, even after treatment with high-dose opioids. To answer this question, Behrends and Larson studied patients who were in severe postoperative pain following surgery who had been treated with intravenous analgesics without pain resolution. A thoracic epidural or peripheral nerve block was placed, and pain relief was obtained with local anesthetic injections. Relief of pain was dramatic without additional opioids. PUAL values and pupil size were unchanged by pain relief (319). Other studies have demonstrated that PUAL is not elevated in patients with severe steady unrelenting postoperative pain compared to other patients with minimal pain. This is not to suggest that acute pain does not dilate the pupil. But the dilation is short-lived, even though the pain from the stimulus continues (320).

When using the PUAL for measurement of opioid effect, it has been observed that heavy sedation and sleep will also diminish PUAL (see Chapter 10; also 220). In addition, the medical record should be examined to ascertain if the patient has evidence of diabetic neuropathy. That condition has been reported to diminish PUAL (321). However, if opioids have been given in doses to nearly ablate PUAL, caution should be taken if regional anesthetics are administered.

In Case Report 12.3, the warning of significant central opioid effect was present with the observation of low PUAL values. This became apparent, however, only after the effect of pain on increasing the respiratory rate was eliminated through the administration of neuraxial block. Thus, steady continuous pain fails to dilate the pupil and augment PUAL values. As the opioid effect intensifies, PUAL will decrease and when this value is below a value of 0.04, then it is unlikely that additional benefit would be obtained with additional opioid therapy, without risking dangerous side effects (310, 317).

Case Report 12.3

A 30-year-old male underwent extensive debridement of leg wounds. Preoperatively, he was a robust male with a remote history of drug abuse, but denied recent ingestion of illicit drugs. On physical examination, he was a normal-appearing male weighing 85 kg with an open draining wound of the left leg. Pupil size was 6.2 mm. Because of prior unpleasant experiences with peripheral nerve blocks and epidural techniques, he preferred general anesthesia, but consented to postoperative epidural analgesia if pain control was difficult to manage in the PACU. In the recovery room, he experienced severe pain arising from the operative site and received large doses of intravenous dilaudid. Nevertheless, he continued to demand additional medication in the PACU. Respiratory rate was 8–10/min and PUAL values near zero. An epidural catheter was placed in the L3–L4 interspace and 8 cc of 2 percent lidocaine injected. Ten minutes later, he was free of pain and became somnolent. Twenty minutes after lidocaine injection, he became unresponsive to verbal and painful stimulation and respiratory rate decreased to 4/min. Oxygen saturation was 88 percent with 5 L/min of nasal oxygen. Positive pressure mask oxygen was delivered, and naloxone 40 mcg was administered intravenously. Within a few minutes, he was fully awake and free of pain. Continuous epidural infusion of dilute bupivacaine with fentanyl then provided satisfactory postoperative analgesia.

Chapter 13

Anisocoria

> Virtue diverse doth a diverse alloyage make with the precious body that it
> quickens, in which, as life in you, it is combined. From the glad nature
> whence it is derived, the mingled virtue through the body shines, even as
> gladness through the living pupil. From these proceeds whatever from light
> to light appeared different, not from dense and rare: This is the formal
> principle that produces, according to its goodness, dark and bright.

(Dante Alighieri, *The Divine Comedy*)

New-onset anisocoria (difference in pupil sizes, right and left) indicates
a disturbance of the natural neurologic symmetry and is therefore abnormal. In
awake patients, the evaluation of anisocoria begins with assessing the pupillary
reactions to increased or decreased ambient light (Figure 13.1; 322–325).
A sympathetic lesion will exhibit an increased difference in pupil sizes in darkness,
whereas a parasympathetic lesion will have increased anisocoria in the light.
Physiological anisocoria is a benign condition that will show the same differences
in pupil size in light or in dark. Both sympathetic and parasympathetic causes of
anisocoria require study by neuro-ophthalmologists because new-onset anisocoria
can indicate serious neuropathology. Algorithms that include topical eye drops and
photographs are often used to locate the cause of anisocoria (323).

The unusual observation of a unilateral dilated pupil during anesthesia is very
concerning to the anesthesia practitioner and can present a disturbing diagnostic
challenge. Although ruptured aneurysms and acute intracranial bleeding can produce anisocoria, other more benign causes are more likely. A rare cause of anisocoria is observed in a patient with long-standing Horner's syndrome that undergoes
a stressful operative procedure. During a case when norepinephrine levels are
elevated, the affected Horner's pupil will dilate to diameters larger than the normal
pupil (Figure 13.2). The details of this case of paradoxical pupillary dilation have
been described (47).

New-onset anisocoria during anesthesia cannot be ignored. Unfortunately, the
diagnostic test using dim and bright light as previously discussed is not useful in
anesthetized patients because the pupils are typically constricted even in darkness.
In addition, new-onset Horner's syndrome cannot be detected during anesthesia
because sympathetic tone in the dilator muscle is not present. Finally, diagnostic
eye drops are not recommended during anesthesia. Use of infrared pupillometry,
however, to evaluate anisocoria during anesthesia can yield valuable information in
a simple and practical way.

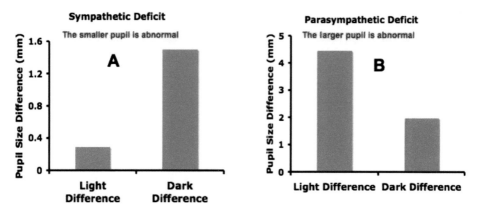

Figure 13.1 In awake patients, the initial test for new-onset anisocoria is to observe the effect of light and dark on the difference in size between the two pupils. A sympathetic lesion similar to Horner's syndrome will exhibit increased anisocoria in dark, but minimal anisocoria in bright light. A parasympathetic lesion that blocks the third nerve will show increased anisocoria in the light. Figure created by the author.

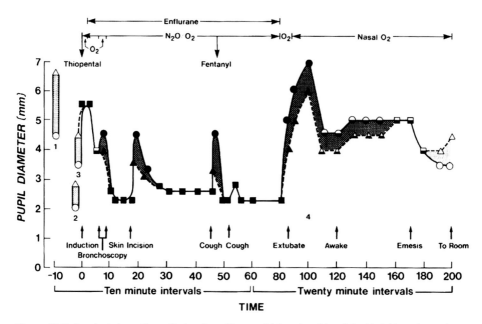

Figure 13.2 Paradoxical pupillary dilation in a 32-year-old female with a left-sided Horner's syndrome undergoing a supraclavicular node biopsy. Left Horner's pupil: circles. Right normal pupil: triangles. During stressful events, the Horner's pupil diameter exceeded the size of the normal pupil. The pupillometer illustrated in Figure 6.1 was used. Subjective estimates of the light reflex are indicated as follows: clear circles and triangles indicate a normal light reflex, filled circles and triangles indicate no light reflex, and partially filled circles and triangles indicate a depressed light reflex. Figure created by author and published in *Anesthesiology Review*, Volume 10, issue 3, March 1983. Journal has been discontinued and permission cannot be obtained.

Case Report 13.1

A 19-year-old developmentally delayed male with asthma and a seizure disorder was scheduled for wisdom tooth extraction. His medications included carbamazepine, loratadine, nasonex, and Atrovent. The patient underwent mask induction with sevoflurane, and received propofol, fentanyl, and rocuronium. His trachea was intubated through the right nostril without complication (no intranasal drugs were used). The anesthesiologist administered intravenous solumedrol and clindamycin and maintained anesthesia with sevoflurane.

The surgeons injected a mixture of 2 percent lidocaine 20 cc, 0.5 percent ropivacaine 10 cc, with 1:100 K epinephrine to block the following nerves: bilateral palatal, bilateral middle superior alveolar, posterior superior alveolar, inferior alveolar, and bilateral buccal. After five teeth were extracted, the anesthesiologist administered neostigmine, glycopyrrolate, ondansetron, and additional fentanyl. Removal of the eye tape revealed a right dilated pupil (8 mm) nonreactive to light, directly and consensually. The left pupil measured 1.5 mm and was reactive to light, both directly and consensually.

The patient's vital signs remained stable throughout the case. After a discussion with senior colleagues and the surgeon regarding potential causes and the possibility of imaging, the senior anesthesiologists elected to awaken the patient. In the PACU, the patient exhibited no mental status changes, but his pupils initially remained anisocoric. After two hours, his pupils returned to 3.5 mm on the left and 3 mm on the right. Both were equally reactive to light directly and consensually. No other ocular abnormalities were noted.

Except in rare situations, where the possibility of pilocarpine eye drops is present in the operating room, the abnormal pupil during anesthesia is the large unreactive pupil. Several case reports have documented a unilateral dilated pupil following inadvertent corneal topical application of atropine, scopolamine, phenylephrine, or cocaine (326–330). These drugs may contact the cornea by hand contamination or via misdirected nasal spray administration. A recent report of anisocoria was discovered to result from contamination of the eye from using underarm Qbrexza topical cloths to prevent sweating (331). Anisocoria from topical agents resolves without sequelae. Diagnosis is made by the realization that these drugs were used for other purposes while near the eye.

Recent reports document a more serious type of complication that is detected by the observation of new-onset anisocoria (332–337). Case Report 13.1 presents a patient who exhibited unilateral anisocoria during general anesthesia that was likely secondary to inadvertent local anesthetic migration directly into the orbital cavity.

Ocular complications following local anesthetic injections for dental surgery have been recently reviewed. Transient blindness, mydriasis, loss of accommodation, and extraocular muscle paralysis have all been reported and result from migration of the local anesthetic into the orbital cavity (338–342). While mydriasis and loss of accommodation would not disturb most patients emerging from general anesthesia, blindness in one eye would be alarming to both the patient and their healthcare providers. It is therefore useful for the clinician to understand and anticipate this potential complication by examining the pupillary light reflex.

As mentioned previously, the standard diagnostic test that is used to diagnose anisocoria in awake subjects cannot be used. Anesthetized patients usually have small pupils, because of concurrent opioid administration, that do not dilate in the dark. It is important to realize in this situation that the "swinging flashlight test" for optic nerve dysfunction (102) (RAPD or relative afferent pupillary defect) will not provide useful information in the anesthetized patient because opioids will prevent significant dilation of the normal pupil when the light is directed into the eye with the afferent defect. However, it is still possible to detect light reflexes with portable infrared pupillometry and this measurement can provide useful information.

The first step is to assess the direct light reflex in the dilated eye. This reflex can be performed with any of the available portable pupillometers using standard techniques. The portable pupillometers can also be used to test the consensual reflex by asking a colleague to illuminate the opposite eye with either a pen light or a cell phone light. In the case study above, there was no direct light reflex in the dilated eye and the eye did not constrict after light was directed into the normal eye. However, light directed into the dilated eye did constrict the pupil of the opposite normal eye.

These tests provided assurance that the optic nerve in the dilated eye was intact. Our case therefore represented local anesthetic blockade of the oculomotor nerve in the orbit without loss of optic nerve function. As a result, the patient was awakened without concern that unilateral blindness would be present on emergence. If both the oculomotor nerve and the optic nerve were blocked, it would seem advisable to wait until the consensual reflex in the normal eye had returned. Optic nerve blockade without involvement of the oculomotor nerve would not result in anisocoria.

Endoscopic sinus surgery can also result in interruption of neural structures within the orbital cavity (343). The medial wall of the orbit is the thinnest of the bony walls of the orbit and is adjacent to the lateral wall of the nasal septum. It is not surprising, therefore, that both the oculomotor and the optic nerves have been injured during these surgical procedures. Because this surgical technique has developed rapidly, it is likely that similar failure of neural transmission within the orbit will be increasingly reported. A review of ophthalmologic complications from endoscopic sinus surgery (337, 343) and case reports of ocular complications during plastic surgery around the eye (344, 345) has verified this prediction. Urgent treatment of optic nerve failure may include intravenous mannitol or acetazolamide, systemic corticosteroids, decompression of the orbit, and topical drugs to lower the intraocular pressure.

Most feared but less common causes of a dilated nonreactive pupil are traumatic and pathologic etiologies, such as traumatic injury, ruptured aneurysms, and other intracranial mass lesions that lead to uncal herniation and compression of the third nerve. However, clinical scenarios must support the possibility of such etiologies. Mechanical trauma in the orbit is unlikely unless the surgeon has accidentally entered the orbit. Significant intraoperative hypertension leading to an intracranial bleed and mass effect could produce a unilateral dilated pupil, but other signs and symptoms would be noted (see Table 13.1 for further discussion).

Table 13.1 is presented to summarize this discussion of new-onset anisocoria during general anesthesia. With a careful review of the case, drugs administered, and attention to the examination of both direct and consensual light reflexes, a diagnosis may frequently be reached without the use of costly imaging procedures (346).

Table 13.1 Diagnosis of new-onset anisocoria during surgical anesthesia

	Affected Pupil Size	Direct Light Reaction of Affected Pupil	Consensual Light Reaction of Affected Pupil	Direct Light Reaction of Unaffected Pupil	Consensual Light Reaction of Unaffected Pupil
Pharmacologic Causes					
Topical Cocaine or Phenylephrine	Large	Low NPi	Low NPi	Normal	Normal
Topical Atropine or Scopolamine	Large	Absent	Absent	Normal	Normal
Local anesthetics injected into orbit (oculomotor blockade only)	Large	Absent	Absent	Normal	Normal
Local anesthetics injected into the orbit (oculomotor & optic nerve blockade)	Large	Absent	Absent	Normal	Absent
Structural Lesions					
Optic nerve trauma during endoscopic sinus surgery	Normal – No Anisocoria	Absent	Normal	Normal	Absent
Oculomotor nerve trauma during endoscopic sinus surgery	Large	Absent	Absent	Normal	Normal
Oculomotor and optic nerve trauma during endoscopic sinus surgery	Large	Absent	Absent	Normal	Absent
Acute trauma or paralysis of dilator sympathetic fibers (acute Horner's)	Normal – No Anisocoria[1]	Normal	Normal	Normal	Normal
Third nerve compression	Large	Absent	Absent	Low NPi[2]	Low NPi

Exam of pupil size and reactivity, both direct and consensual, can help in identifying an etiology of new-onset anisocoria during anesthesia. The term "sluggish" pupil is a clinical impression that has never been defined. It is more appropriate to quantify the reaction of the pupil with an objective infrared pupillometer. Small miotic pupils are difficult to assess with the simple pen-light examination.

[1] The dilator muscle has no sympathetic tone in anesthetized subjects, so the anisocoria of Horner's syndrome is not present during anesthesia (13, 99). Patients with Horner's syndrome prior to surgery may exhibit paradoxical dilation of the sympathectomized pupil following the skin incision (47).

[2] A historical analysis of the case is essential when considering this diagnosis. It should be considered when other causes listed in the table have been eliminated. Increased intracranial pressure will also produce an abnormal light reflex in the smaller pupil, detected with pupillometry (250). Dilute pilocarpine (1 percent) will constrict the dilated pupil with third nerve compression, but will have no effect on the dilated pupil secondary to muscarinic blocking agents (76). The dilated Adie's pupil discussed in Chapter 5 will constrict to very dilute concentrations of pilocarpine (0.1 percent) because it has developed denervation supersensitivity to acetylcholine (76, 283).

Approval was granted to J. G. Broch-Utne to publish the above chart in his book, *Case Studies of Near Misses in Clinical Anesthesia*, Springer, 2011.

Case Reports

My son, obey my words, and treasure my commands. Keep my commands and live; protect my teachings as the pupil of your eye. Tie them to your fingers; write them on the tablet of your heart.

(*The Holy Bible*, Proverbs)

A statistical analysis of observational studies that include hundreds of cases cannot define the value of pupillometry for any one case. Physicians deal with one case at a time. Whatever information can be obtained from laboratory tests and other physiological values along with pupillometry can help decide on the condition of that patient. The following case reports are examples of how pupillometry has benefitted case management. The author does not imply that the following cases could not have been managed without pupillometry. However, pupillary measurements did reveal timely information about the condition of each patient.

One recent published case report described a patient with bilateral absent light reflexes on visual inspection (347). This patient was spared surgery when an infrared pupillometer revealed that pupil reactivity was present. In a separate study, an analysis of 16 clinically absent light reflexes while using a pen light revealed intact reflexes in 25 percent of these cases using infrared pupillometry. In this study of comatose patients, a dark iris with a dilated pupil was often mistaken as having no light reflex that was detected as present with infrared pupillometry (Figure 14.1; 348).

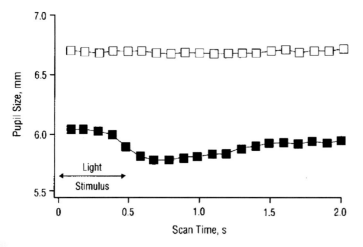

Figure 14.1 Top tracing: Averaged pupillometric scans from confirmed brain-dead subjects. Bottom tracing: Averaged pupillometric scans from patients who were reported to have absent light reflexes. Portable infrared pupillometers can often record light reflexes in patients whose reflexes are reported absent with the traditional pen-light examination. Permission to reproduce image from *JAMA Neurology*. License Number: 5627661465787.

The following case reports expand on this idea by describing how the pupillometer provided information to the author and his colleagues that was useful to clinical management. These cases are selected from the author's own practice as an attending physician in a tertiary hospital with complex surgical procedures and frequent calls for airway assistance during cardiopulmonary resuscitation. They do not represent the diverse applications of portable pupillometry in other medical specialties. The pupillary measurements were simply one test out of many that helped us to understand the condition of the patient. No identifying features of these cases were retained, and consents were secured from patients who survived.

Case Report 14.1

A 45-year-old, 66 kg female was operated for a left temporal–parietal meningioma. The procedure was performed in the semi-lateral position with propofol, isoflurane, nitrous oxide, and muscle relaxants. A lumbar drain was placed during the procedure and 30 cc of CSF was withdrawn intraoperatively. This drain was removed before transfer to the PACU. On the second postoperative day, the patient exhibited increasing lethargy, anisocoria, and an absent pupillary light reflex on the left, with preserved reflexes on the right. Computerized axial tomography demonstrated a left temporal–parietal epidural hematoma together with uncal herniation and she was emergently scheduled for evacuation of an epidural hematoma. The procedure was completed without significant blood loss, hypotension, or hypoxic episodes. Because of concern for postoperative edema and increased intracranial pressure, the bone flap was not replaced. She remained obtunded following surgery and was left intubated overnight, but was extubated the following morning after demonstrating full voluntary motor strength and adequate gag reflexes. However, the following day, she was observed to be obtunded again, with absent pupillary light reflex on the left, and reduced reflexes on the right. An endotracheal tube was placed, and she returned to surgery for a wide excision of the tentorium. She remained intubated overnight and was then extubated the following morning while fully awake and following commands. For the next two days, she remained in the intensive care unit because of failure to maintain consciousness in the sitting position. While supine, she was alert and intact, but within 20 minutes of sitting upright, she developed lethargy, which quickly proceeded to loss of consciousness and return of abnormal pupillary reflexes. After two days of this unusual syndrome, an epidural blood patch was performed with 30 cc of blood introduced into the L2–L3 epidural space. Four hours later, she was placed in the upright position and her mental state and pupillary reflexes were unchanged for 25 minutes (251).

In consultation with the neurosurgeons, it was suggested that the development of abnormal pupillary reflexes in the sitting position was a result of uncal herniation, partially secondary to a CSF leak from the lumbar drain puncture. This was confirmed by the observation that her pupillary reflexes remained normal, and her mental state did not deteriorate after placement of a blood patch.

Case Report 14.2

A 74-year-old male was undergoing debridement of leg ulcers with isoflurane, fentanyl, and oxygen anesthesia. During closure of the surgical wounds, the anesthetic concentrations were lowered, but the patient moved, and the subsequent coughing and straining led to the administration of a propofol bolus and an increase in the isoflurane concentration. Following return of immobility, heart rate from the EKG monitor was 65, but no blood pressure could be obtained, and no pulse was detected. CPR was begun immediately and 50–100 mcg bolus injections of epinephrine were administered. The blood pressure returned briefly, and an arterial line was inserted into the radial artery. Within 3 minutes, the blood pressure became unobtainable, but the EKG was unchanged. CPR was reinstituted and epinephrine bolus injections and a continuous infusion of epinephrine of 10 mcg/min and atropine 1 mg were administered. CPR continued for another 20 minutes, before blood pressure again returned and was stabilized with dopamine and epinephrine infusions. Throughout the resuscitation, pupil size and light reflex were measured with a portable infrared pupillometer. After the circulation was restored, the normal light reflex returned within 3 minutes. The light reflex returned before there was any movement, swallowing, or coughing. Following insertion of a pulmonary catheter, the patient was transferred to the ICU. He began to awaken within 2 hours and was ready for extubation within 4 hours. Because of the uncertain nature of the arrest, he was sedated and ventilated for the next 12 hours while diagnostic tests were analyzed. Return of neurologic function was complete and he was discharged from the hospital on the fourth postoperative day.

The rapid return of the light reflex soon after ROSC was a reassuring sign that brain stem function was not irreversibly damaged. The case also demonstrates that large doses of atropine and epinephrine do not block the light reflex, a finding that has been confirmed by subsequent authors (268).

Case Report 14.3

A 19-year-old male underwent correction of pectus excavatum. An epidural catheter was inserted in the T7–T8 interspace before induction of anesthesia. The catheter tested negative for intravascular and intrathecal positions. The early portion of the anesthetic was conducted with remifentanil, isoflurane, and nitrous oxide/oxygen. During closure, incremental doses of 0.5 percent bupivacaine were administered via the epidural catheter and simultaneously the remifentanil was discontinued. As the remifentanil effect dissipated, the segmental nature of the resulting epidural block became apparent. Intermittent testing at the two stimulating sites initially revealed complete blockade of PRD at T4, but dilations at C3. As the dressings were applied, a movable electrode demonstrated that the block was complete two segments above the incision. The hemodynamic changes during the transition period in this case were confusing. Blood pressure and heart rate both increased as the effects of remifentanil dissipated.

This case demonstrates that blood pressure and heart rate are not always accurate measures of a functioning epidural. Testing of different sites with sterile EKG pads confirmed that the epidural would provide segmental analgesia during emergence and that administration of additional opioids would be unnecessary.

Case Report 14.4

A 45-year-old 43 kg female was scheduled for excision of a mass of the left shoulder. After a discussion of the options for anesthetic management, she elected to have general anesthesia, in combination with an interscalene nerve block. Twenty-five cc of 0.5 percent bupivacaine was injected into the left interscalene groove with ultrasound guidance. Immediately following the injection, she was anesthetized with propofol 100 mg, 100 mcg fentanyl, and desflurane at 4 percent end-tidal. Tracheal intubation was assisted by administration of 5 mg vecuronium. Following positioning of the patient by the surgical team and at 18 minutes after injection of bupivacaine, EKG pads were placed over the site of the anticipated incision on the left shoulder and onto the corresponding area of the right shoulder. Alternative stimulation of both sites 20 minutes after injection revealed a total lack of pupillary dilation following stimulation of the left shoulder, but a 1.5 mm dilation from the right shoulder. Minimal anesthetic agents were used during the procedure, and she was awakened 2.5 hours later with complete analgesia of the operative site.

Case Report 14.5

Buprenorphine is an unusual mu-opioid agonist that is commonly used to treat opioid abuse disorder. It is a weak agonist, but binds tightly to the mu receptor. It has the property of partially blocking the more profound analgesic effects of the stronger mu agonists, such as morphine. The following case report used pupillometry to demonstrate that neither postoperative pain nor PUAL were decreased with morphine in a patient taking buprenorphine.

A 64-year-old male presented for open right partial nephrectomy. He was taking Suboxone 8 mg twice daily. Preoperative PUAL values were within the range of normal for his age. Postoperatively, after increasing the dose of Suboxone, escalating doses of morphine from 60 to 200 mg in 24 hours failed to affect either pain scores or PUAL values (Figure 14.2). Lidoderm patches, relaxation therapy, and warm packs were added, which resulted in acceptable pain scores. He was discharged from the hospital on his original dose of Suboxone to be followed by his Pain Clinic.

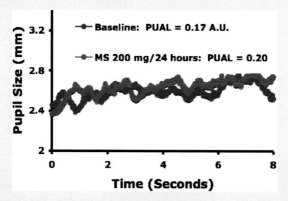

Figure 14.2 Pupillary unrest was not diminished, and pain was not controlled by administration of morphine in this postoperative patient taking Suboxone.
Pupillometry readings taken from a consenting patient.

Case Report 14.6

A 13-month-old male child was undergoing insertion of a Broviac catheter with sevo-flurane, fentanyl, and oxygen. Shortly following insertion of the subclavian needle, the heart rate taken from the EKG monitor increased from 100 to 118, the noninvasive blood pressure monitor recorded an error message, and the pulse oximeter was in search mode. A pulse was thought to be present in the neck. Numerous attempts were made to read the blood pressure and obtain a pulse oximeter reading. The circulating nurse called for another anesthesiologist who, upon arrival, noted 5 mm nonreactive pupils and low end-tidal CO_2 values. CPR was instituted and the chest was rapidly opened. A large amount of blood was evacuated from the pleural cavity. A puncture wound of the subclavian artery was noted and repair was attempted, while the patient was volume resuscitated and open cardiac massage was begun. Despite vigorous resuscitation attempts, the EKG deteriorated to an agonal rhythm and the patient died on the table.

Electromechanical dissociation can persist for several minutes after cardiac output has dropped to zero. The pupil begins to dilate within several seconds after cardiac arrest. It is possible that a rapid appreciation of the 5-mm nonreactive pupil in this case may have resulted in a more timely resuscitation effort.

Case Report 14.7

A 61-year-old 81 kg female (BMI 41) was scheduled for hysterectomy and lymph node dissection for carcinoma of the uterus. She was hypertensive and had coronary artery disease requiring stent placements within the past year. Her medications, taken also on the morning of admission, included atenolol and lisinopril. An epidural catheter was positioned in the T9–T10 interspace, and a test dose of lidocaine and epinephrine was negative. Twelve ml of 0.5 percent ropivacaine was injected through the epidural catheter. Anesthesia was induced with propofol and sevoflurane and following adminis-tration of 50 mg of rocuronium, the trachea was intubated. Testing of the T10 dermatome was begun 20 minutes after injection of ropivacaine and revealed persistent pupillary dilations following 100 milliamps of current through surface EKG pads. The skin incision produced marked pupillary dilation, with no change in heart rate or blood pressure. The case proceeded without incident. Antinociception during emergence was achieved with intravenous fentanyl instead of epidural local anesthetics. The epidural catheter was removed after extubation of the trachea.

This case is another example of how reliance on the blood pressure and heart rate response to incision is a poor indicator of the adequacy of the epidural block. Antihypertensive medications can block the effect of nociception on blood pressure and heart rate.

Case Report 14.8

An 82-year-old male was found to be unresponsive 8 days after extensive surgery for lumbar and thoracic spine disease. The code blue team was called for evaluation and resuscitation. Upon arrival, the patient was apneic, had 3-mm reactive pupils, and was not following commands. Opioids and benzodiazepines had been administered prior to the code. Blood pressure was 80/50 and heart rate was 70. Naloxone 0.8 mg was administered without effect. Pupils remained at 3.0 mm bilaterally and the patient did not move. Intubation of the trachea was performed without relaxants, and he was transferred to the intensive care unit. An MRI of the spine revealed an extensive epidural hematoma extending throughout the thoracic and cervical spine, with compression of the brain stem. Evacuation of the hematoma was performed that day with a gradual return of consciousness and residual weakness of both arms.

Pupillometry suggested that the small pupils in this case were unrelated to opioid administration and a suspected bilateral Horner's syndrome was a possible diagnosis. Thus, in suspected opioid overdose, an aberrant pupil is one that does not dilate in response to naloxone. The cause of apnea may be unrelated to opioid overdose and other causes should then be suspected.

Case Report 14.9

A T7–T8 epidural catheter was placed in a 58-year-old female scheduled for a partial hepatectomy. Test dose was negative, and she was induced with propofol, rocuronium, and esmolol. Oral intubation was performed and sevoflurane and 80 percent oxygen were administered. The resident attached the epidural infusion line of 0.2 percent ropivacaine to the epidural catheter and then "programmed" the pump to deliver 10 cc of the epidural solution into the epidural space. The anesthetic team then directed their attention to other activities such as antibiotic administration, time out, insertion of arterial lines, and a CVP. Blood pressure was observed to be 70 systolic, but responded rapidly to bolus injections and a continuous infusion of phenylephrine. As the drapes were applied, the resident observed that the epidural pump was still infusing local anesthetic into the epidural space. When this was noticed, 75 cc of 0.2 percent bupivacaine had already been delivered. An infusion of phenylephrine had already been initiated and the condition of the patient was unremarkable. Testing for pupillary dilation over the C3 dermatome resulted in no change in pupil size, whereas a tetanic stimulus delivered from electrodes positioned on the mandible exhibited a brisk dilation. The epidural infusion was discontinued and not restarted until the pupil started to dilate during the surgical procedure.

Pupillometry in this case confirmed the presence of total epidural blockade. Additionally, it was noted that the block eventually receded into dermatomes appropriate for the surgery.

Case Report 14.10

A 32-year-old male was taking methadone daily each morning for chronic pain resulting from a motorcycle accident 8 years prior to admission. He was admitted for pain control that was exacerbated by a minor acute injury to his chronically painful right leg that had been amputated below the knee. The methadone clinic administered the drug once per day in a dose of 300 mg at 9 am daily and the clinic wanted to maintain once-per-day dosing of opioids while in the hospital. Adjuvant analgesics were started that included Tylenol, ketamine, and diclofenac. PUAL and pupil size were measured at 8 am, 30 minutes prior to his morning dose of methadone. At that time, he was in pain and unable to eat breakfast. His PUAL value was unusually high at 0.57 AU. Two hours after methadone treatment and IV dilaudid, his PUAL had decreased, and he was eating and reported 3/10 pain. Although adjuvant non-opioid drugs were given, he was once again in pain 6 hours after the methadone. He was resigned to the fact that our supplemental therapy was not effective, and he would have to endure his pain until the following morning. The clinical picture in this case was an incipient opioid withdrawal every morning prior to his daily methadone dose. A noticeable pattern prior to his early morning methadone dose was high-amplitude, low-frequency fluctuations that were unrelated to acute painful stimulation of the affected limb. In this case, dose adjustments were made to satisfy the patient's pain therapy. Similar patterns have been observed in other subjects during incipient opioid withdrawal (Figure 14.3). On the other hand, a small pupil with low PUAL scores in a patient with significant postoperative pain signifies that the benefit of systemic opioids has been maximized and other methods of pain control are indicated (326).

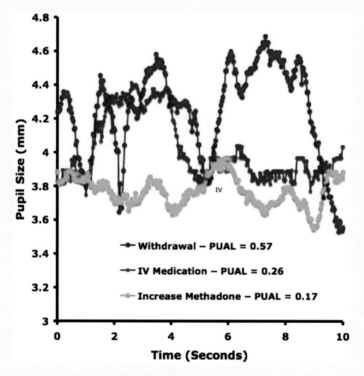

Figure 14.3 PUAL varies from subject to subject. Wide fluctuations in pupil size suggest opioid withdrawal that can be confirmed by other physical signs.
Pupillometry measurements taken from a consenting patient.

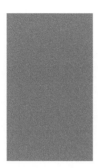

Conclusion

He had a curious gift. He was able to fix his eyes upon you for an immensely long time, and the glassy stare of them, with their dilated pupils was simply terrifying.

(W. Somerset Maugham, *Christmas Holiday*)

He sustained them in a desert land
In an empty howling wasteland
He encompassed them and raised them up,
Protecting them like the pupil of his eye.

(*The Holy Bible*, Deuteronomy 32:10)

Portable pupillometry is expanding rapidly in clinical and research settings (167, 182, 224, 232, 242, 259, 263, 275, 280, 297, 349–361). Over 10,000 references with the subject pupillometry are listed in Medline Central for the past 10 years. Many of these references relate to measurement of the pupil with desktop computers or with head-mounted goggles. Portable pupillometry that can be used in the hospital or office setting comprises a significant number of recent publications on pupillometry. The possibility of expanding portable pupillometry into mobile phone applications is under study. Instruments are becoming more user friendly and now retrieve accurate information that is impossible to obtain with the traditional pen-light examination.

The portable instruments are now easier to use, but to make meaningful measurements they must be taken consistently. A trend of the size of the pupil lacks relevance if sequential measurements are taken in different light settings and with variable techniques.

The measurement of the pupil is useless if it cannot be interpreted. Some basic understanding of the physiology of the pupil is essential to make the reflexes useful. For example, some patients with tonic pupils have no reflexes. This occurrence is rare, but knowledge of these various rare syndromes is essential when any pupillary reflexes are evaluated. The references listed below contain information that will assist in the interpretation of the pupillary measurements. Finally, if the pupil has information that might assist the clinician, then accurate measurements are essential. Lord Kelvin was one of the prominent scientists of the late nineteenth century and his contributions to the scientific literature could have never been made without accurate measurements. In his own words: "when you cannot measure it, your knowledge is of a meager and unsatisfactory kind" (362).

References

1. JC Eccles, RM Eccles, A Iggo, A Lundberg. Electrophysiological investigations on Renshaw cells. *J Physiol.* 1961; 1593: 461–78.

2. RM Eccles. Inhibition by Renshaw's cells. *Actual Neurophysiol Paris.* 1962; 4: 55–66.

3. EJ Walaszek, JE Chapman. Bulbocapnine: An adrenergic and serotonin blocking agent. J *Pharmacol Exp Ther.* 1962; 137: 285–90.

4. RG Pendleton, E Finlay, S Sherman. Effect of bulbocapine as a peripheral dopamine receptor antagonist in the anesthetized cat. *Naunyn Schmiedebergs Arch Pharmacol.* 1975; 289: 171–8.

5. FF Weight, GC Salmoiraghi. Adrenergic responses of Renshaw cells. *J Pharmacol Exp Ther.* 1966; 154: 391–7.

6. F Bremer. Cerveau "isole" et physiologie du sommeil. *Compte Rendus de la Société de Biologie Paris.* 1935; 118: 1235–45.

7. MD Larson. An analysis of the action of strychnine on the recurrent IPSP and amino acid induced inhibitions in the cat spinal cord. *Brain Res.* 1969; 15: 185–200.

8. MD Larson, MA Major. The effect of hexobarbital on the duration of the recurrent IPSP in cat motoneurons. *Brain Res.* 1970; 212: 309–11.

9. AE Guedel. *Inhalation Anesthesia.* New York: Macmillan; 1937, pp. 1–140.

10. J Poe. The eye signs and their significance in general anesthesia. *Curr Res Anesth Analgesia.* 1926; 5: 156–9.

11. DJ Cullen, EI Eger, 2nd, WC Stevens, NT Smith, TH Cromwell, BF Cullen, et al. Clinical signs of anesthesia. *Anesthesiology.* 1972; 36: 21–36.

12. J Posner, CB Saper, ND Schiff, J Classen. *Plum and Posner's Diagnosis and Treatment of Stupor and Come.* New York: Oxford University Press; 2019.

13. IE Loewenfeld. Mechanism of reflex dilation of the pupil: Historical review and experimental analysis. *Doc Opthalmol.* 1958; 12: 184–448.

14. HK Lee, SC Wang. Mechanism of morphine-induced miosis in the dog. *J Pharmacol Exp Ther.* 1975; 192: 415–31.

15. MD Larson. Pupillary effects of general anesthesia. *Anesthesiol Rev.* 1986; 13: 25–31.

16. L Stark. The pupillary control system: Its non-linear adaptive and stochastic engineering design characteristics. *Automatica.* 1969; 5: 655–76.

17. MD Larson, DI Sessler, J McGuire, JM Hynson. Isoflurane, but not mild hypothermia, depresses the human pupillary light reflex. *Anesthesiology.* 1991; 75: 62–7.

18. MD Larson, DI Sessler, DE Washington, BR Merrifield, JA Hynson, J McGuire. Pupillary response to noxious stimulation during isoflurane and propofol anesthesia. *Anesth Analg.* 1993; 76: 1072–8.

19. L Da Vinci. *Codex Arundel.* The British Library: 1478–1519.

20. DS Strong. *Leonardo on the Eye: A Critical Commentary of Manuscript D in the Bibliotheque Nationale.* Paris: Self Published; 1979.

21. CD Yic, G Prada, SI Paz, L Moraes, JC Pontet, ME Lasso, et al. Comparison of ultrasonographic versus infrared pupillary assessment. *Ultrasound J.* 2020; 12: 38.

22. NJ Volpe, ES Plotkin, MG Maguire, R Hariprasad, SL Galetta. Portable pupillography of the swinging flashlight test to detect afferent pupillary defects. *Ophthalmology.* 2000; 107: 1913–21.

23. HS Thompson. The vitality of the pupil: A history of the clinical use of the pupil as

an indicator of visual potential. *J Neuro-ophthalmol.* 2003; 23: 213–24.

24. KW Ascher. The first pupillary light reflex test ever performed. *Trans Am Ophthalmol Soc.* 1962; 60: 53–9.

25. KW Ascher. The first test of the pupillary reflex to light. *Boll Ocul.* 1963; 42: 586–91.

26. NJ Wade, S Finger. The eye as an optical instrument: From camera obscura to Helmholtz's perspective. *Perception.* 2001; 30: 1157–77.

27. R Whytt. *An Essay on the Vital and Other Involuntary Motions of Animals.* Edinburgh: T. Beckert, Auld & Smellie; 1751.

28. R Whytt. *The Works of Robert Whytt.* Edinburgh: T. Beckert, Auld & Smellie ; 1768.

29. A Kolliker. Ueber den Dilatator Pupillae. *Anat Anz.* 1897; 154.

30. M Hall. On the reflex function of the medulla oblongata and the medulla spinalis. *Phil Trans Roy Soc Lond.* 1833; 1833: 635–65.

31. F Fontana. Dei moti dell'iride. *Nella Stamp Jacopo Giusti.* 1765; 1–106.

32. J Mery. Des mouvements de l'iris, et par occasion, de lar partie principale de l'organe de la vue. *Histoire Académie Roy Sci Paris.* 1704; 261–71.

33. P de la Hire. Explication de quelques faits d'optique and de la manière dont se fait la vision. *Mem Acad Roy Sci.* 1709; 119–32.

34. A Haller. *A Dissertation on the Sensible and Irritable Parts of Animals.* London: Gottingae; 1755.

35. E Weber, EH Weber. Ecperiments on galvanomaneticae irritatos, motum cordis retardare et adeo intercipare. *Ann Univ Med Milano.* 1845; 20: 227–33.

36. CS Sherrington. *The Integrative Action of the Nervous System.* New Haven, CT: Yale University Press; 1906.

37. L Brock, J Coombs, J Eccles. The recording of potentials from motoneurones with an intracellular electrode. *J Physiol.* 1952; 117: 431–60.

38. GF Rossi. Study of the nature of miosis during sleep and during barbiturate anesthesia. *Arch Sci Biol.* 1957; 41: 46–56.

39. IE Loewenfeld. *The Pupil: Anatomy, Physiology and Clinical Applications.* Woburn, MA: Butterworth-Heinemann; 1999.

40. C Peinkhofer, GM Knudsen, R Moretti, D Kondziella. Cortical modulation of pupillary function: Systematic review. *Peer J.* 2019; e6882.

41. R Knox. *An Historical Account of the Island of Ceylon in the East Indies.* London: Robert Chiswell; 1681.

42. CR Keeler. 150 years since Babbage's ophthalmoscope. *Arch Ophthalmol.* 1997; 115: 1456–7.

43. HL Helmholtz. *Beschreibung eines Augen-Spiefels zur Intersuchung der Netzhaut im lebenden Auge.* Berlin: Forstner; 1851.

44. ES Gifford. *The Evil Eye.* New York: The MacMillan Co.; 1958.

45. F-P du Petit. Mémoire dans laquelle il est démontré que les nerfs intercostaux fournissent des rameaux qui portent des espirits dans les yeux. *Mem Acad Sci.* 1727; 1–19.

46. HK Anderson. Paradoxical pupillary dilation and other ocular phenomena caused by lesions of the cervical sympathetic tract. *J Physiol.* 1903; 30: 290–310.

47. MD Larson, CA Gibbons, FKM Chiu. Paradoxical pupillary dilation in a patient with Horner's syndrome. *Anesthesiol Rev.* 1983; 10: 22–5.

48. WB Cannon, A Rosenblueth. *Supersensitivity of Denervated Structures.* New York: Macmillan; 1949.

49. PD Gamlin, DH McDougal, J Pokorny, VC Smith, KW Yau, DM Dacey. Human and macaque pupil responses driven by melanopsin-containing retinal ganglion cells. *Vision Res.* 2007; 47: 946–54.

50. L Edinger. Ueber enn Verlauf der centralen Hirnnervenbahnen mit Demonstration von Praparaten. *Archiv Psychiatrie Nervenkrankheiten.* 1885; 16: 858–89.

51. CFO Westphal. Ueber einen Fall von chronischer progressiver Lahmung der Augenmuskeln. *Archiv Psychiatrie Nervenkrankheiten.* 1887; 18: 846–71.

52. A Zuniga, AE Ryabinin. Involvement of centrally projecting Edinger-Westphal nucleus neuropeptides in actions of addictive drugs. *Brain Sci.* 2020; 10: 2.

53. T Kozicz, JC Bittencourt, PJ May, A Reiner, PD Gamlin, M Palkovits, et al. The Edinger-Westphal nucleus: A historical, structural, and functional perspective on a dichotomous terminology. *J Comp Neurol.* 2011; 519: 1413–34.

54. PJ May, W Sun, NF Wright, JT Erichsen. Pupillary light reflex circuits in the macaque monkey: The preganglionic Edinger-Westphal nucleus. *Brain Struct Funct.* 2020; 225: 403–25.

55. AM Sillito, AW Zbrozyna. The activity characteristics of the preganglionic pupilloconstrictor neurones. *J Physiol.* 1970; 211: 767–79.

56. MD Larson, M Behrends. Portable infrared pupillometry: A review. *Anesth Analg.* 2015; 120: 1242–53.

57. MD Larson, DI Sessler, DE Washington, BR Merrifield, JA Hynson, J McGuire. Pupillary response to noxious stimulation during isoflurane and propofol anesthesia. *Anesth Analg.* 1993; 76: 1072–8.

58. H Eilers, MD Larson. The effect of ketamine and nitrous oxide on the human pupillary light reflex during general anesthesia. *Auton Neurosci.* 2010; 152: 108–14.

59. AV Rukmini, D Milea, JJ Gooley. Chromatic pupillometry methods for assessing photoreceptor health in retinal and optic nerve diseases. *Front Neurol.* 2019; 10: 76.

60. LS Mure. Intrinsically photosensitive retinal ganglion cells of the human retina. *Front Neurol.* 2021; 12: 636330.

61. J Zeitzer, R Najjar, M Kass. Impact of blue-depleted white light on pupil dynamics, melatonin suppression and subjective alertness following real-world light exposure. *Sleep Sci Pract.* 2018; 1: 1–23.

62. S Mathot. Pupillometry: Psychology, physiology, and function. *J Cogn.* 2018; 11: 16.

63. AJ Zele, PD Gamlin. Editorial: The pupil: Behavior, anatomy, physiology and clinical biomarkers. *Front Neurol.* 2020; 11: 211.

64. SR Steinhauer, R Condray, A Kasparek. Cognitive modulation of midbrain function: Task-induced reduction of the pupillary light reflex. *Int J Psychophysiol.* 2000; 39: 21–30.

65. SR Steinhauer, G Hakerem. The pupillary response in cognitive psychophysiology and schizophrenia. *Ann N Y Acad Sci.* 1992; 658: 182–204.

66. SR Steinhauer, G Hakerem, BJ Spring. The pupillary response as a potential indicator of vulnerability to schizophrenia. *Psychopharmacol Bull.* 1979; 15: 44–5.

67. SR Steinhauer, MM Bradley, GJ Siegle, KA Roecklein, A Dix. Publication guidelines and recommendations for pupillary measurement in psychophysiological studies. *Psychophysiology.* 2022; 59: e14035.

68. C Kelbsch, T Strasser, Y Chen, B Feigl, PD Gamlin, R Kardon, et al. Standards in pupillography. *Front Neurol.* 2019; 10: 129.

69. C Citrenbaum, J Corlier, D Ngo, N Vince-Cruz, A Wilson, SA Wilke, et al. Pretreatment pupillary reactivity is associated with differential early response to 10 Hz and intermittent theta-burst repetitive transcranial magnetic stimulation (rTMS) treatment of major depressive disorder (MDD). *Brain Stimul.* 2023; 6: 1566–71.

70. MH Papesh, SD Goldinger (eds). *Modern Pupillometry: Cognition, Neuroscience, and Practical Applications.* New York: Springer International; 2024.

71. JC Eccles. The synapse: From electrical to chemical transmission. *Annu Rev Neurosci.* 1982; 5: 325–39.

72. F Glisson. *Anatomia Hepatis.* London: Du-Gard for Pullein; 1654.

73. TR Elliott. On the action of adrenalin. *Proceedings of the Physiological Society of London*; May 21, 1904.

74. O Loewi. On the background of the discovery of neurochemical transmission. *J Mt Sinai Hosp New York.* 1957; 24: 1014–16.

75. J Bernstein. Zer Irisbewegung. Erwiderung an Herrn Grunhagen. *Z Rat Med.* 1867; 29: 35–7.

76. FD Bremner. The fixed dilated pupil. Pilocarpine better than a scan. *Br Med J.* 2008; 336: 171.

77. MD Larson. A simple test for scopolamine mydriasis. *Anesth Analg.* 1991; 73: 824.

78. A Proudfoot. The early toxicology of physostigmine: A tale of beans, great men and egos. *Toxicol Rev.* 2006; 25: 99–138.

79. JL Langley, HK Anderson. On the mechanisms of the movements of the iris. *J Physiol.* 1892; 13: 500–97.

80. MB Bender, EA Weinstein. Actions of adrenalin and acetylcholine on the denervated iris of the cat and monkey. *Am J Physiol.* 1940; 130: 268–75.

81. R Omary, CJ Bockisch, K Landau, RH Kardon, KP Weber. Buzzing sympathetic nerves: A new test to enhance anisocoria in Horner's syndrome. *Front Neurol.* 2019; 10: 107.

82. JN Langley. Sketch of the progress of discovery in the eighteenth century as regards the autonomic nervous system. *J Physiol.* 1916; 504: 225–58.

83. JN Langley. On the stimulation and paralysis of nerve cells and nerve endings: Part II. Paralysis by curari, strychnine and brucine and its antagonism by nicotine. *J Physiol.* 1918; 52: 247–66.

84. JN Langley. The vascular dilatation caused by the sympathetic and the course of vaso-motor nerves. *J Physiol.* 1923; 58: 70–3.

85. WD Paton. The paralysis of autonomic ganglia, with special reference to the therapeutic effect of ganglion-blocking drugs. *Br Med J.* 1951; 1: 773–8.

86. U Erdem, FC Gundogan, UA Dinc, U Yolcu, A Ilhan, S Altun. Acute effect of cigarette smoking on pupil size and ocular aberrations: A pre- and post-smoking study. *J Ophthalmol.* 2015; 625470.

87. RJ Roberge, EP Krenzelok. Prolonged coma and loss of brainstem reflexes following amitriptyline overdose. *Vet Hum Toxicol.* 2001; 43: 42–4.

88. MD Larson, PO Talke. Effect of dexmedetomidine, an alpha2-adrenoceptor agonist, on human pupillary reflexes during general anaesthesia. *Br J Clin Pharmacol.* 2001; 51: 27–33.

89. MD Larson. The effect of antiemetics on pupillary reflex dilation during epidural/general anesthesia. *Anesth Analg.* 2003; 97: 1652–6.

90. JL Pretorius, M Phillips, RW Langley, E Szabadi, CM Bradshaw. Comparison of clozapine and haloperidol on some autonomic and psychomotor functions, and on serum prolactin concentration, in healthy subjects. *Br J Clin Pharmacol.* 2001; 52: 322–6.

91. CP Campobasso, F De Micco, G Corbi, T Keller, B Hartung, T Daldrup, et al. Pupillary effects in habitual cannabis consumers quantified with pupillography. *Forensic Sci Int.* 2020; 317: 110559.

92. RL Hartman, JE Richman, CE Hayes, MA Huestis. Drug Recognition Expert (DRE) examination characteristics of cannabis impairment. *Accid Anal Prev.* 2016; 92: 219–29.

93. EA Kolbrich, RS Goodwin, DA Gorelick, RJ Hayes, EA Stein, MA Huestis. Physiological and subjective responses to controlled oral 3,4-methylenedioxymethamphetamine administration. *J Clin Psychopharmacol.* 2008; 28: 432–40.

94. ST Charles, DI Hamasaki. The effect of intraocular pressure on the pupil size. *Arch Ophthalmol.* 1970; 83: 729–33.

95. AA Siddiqui, JC Clarke, A Grzybowski. William John Adie: The man behind the syndrome. *Clin Exp Ophthalmol.* 2014; 42: 778–84.

96. S Bista Karki, KJ Coppell, LV Mitchell, KC Ogbuehi. Dynamic pupillometry in type 2 diabetes: Pupillary autonomic dysfunction and the severity of diabetic retinopathy. *Clin Ophthalmol.* 2020; 14: 3923–30.

97. DM Levy, DA Rowley, RR Abraham. Portable infrared pupillometry using Pupilscan: Relation to somatic and autonomic nerve function in diabetes mellitus. *Clin Auton Res.* 1992; 2: 335–41.

98. GL Ferrari, JL Marques, RA Gandhi, SR Heller, FK Schneider, S Tesfaye, et al. Using dynamic pupillometry as a simple screening tool to detect autonomic neuropathy in patients with diabetes: A pilot study. *Biomed Eng Online.* 2010; 9: 26.

99. MD Larson, F Tayefeh, DI Sessler, M Daniel, M Noorani. Sympathetic nervous system does not mediate reflex pupillary dilation during desflurane anesthesia. *Anesthesiology.* 1996; 85: 748–54.

100. EI Eger, RB Weiskopf. Sympathetic hyperactivity during desflurane anesthesia. *Anesthesiology.* 1994; 80: 482–3.

101. MD Larson, WC Herman. Bilateral dilated nonreactive pupils during surgery in a patient with undiagnosed pheochromocytoma. *Anesthesiology.* 1992; 77: 200–2.

102. P Levatin. Pupillary escape in disease of the retina or optic nerve. *Arch Ophthalmol.* 1959; 62: 768–79.

103. RK Talukder, SR Sutradhar, KM Rahman, MJ Uddin, H Akhter. Guillain-Barré syndrome. *Mymensingh Med J.* 2011; 20: 748–56.

104. B Kaymakamzade, F Selcuk, A Koysuren, AI Colpak, SE Mut, T Kansu. Pupillary involvement in Miller Fisher Syndrome. *Neuro-Ophthalmology.* 2013; 37: 111–15.

105. J Liu, F Tang, X Chen, Z Li. Guillain-Barré syndrome with incomplete oculomotor nerve palsy after traumatic brain injury: Case report and literature review. *Brain Sci.* 2023; 13: 527.

106. MD Larson. Dilation of the pupil in human subjects after intravenous thiopental. *Anesthesiology.* 1981; 54: 246–9.

107. MJF Ravnborg, NH Jensen, IK Holk. Pupillary diameter and ventilatory carbon dioxide sensitivity after epidural morphine and buprenorphine in volunteers. *Anesth Analg.* 1987; 66: 847–51.

108. MD Larson. Alteration of the human pupillary light reflex by general anesthesia. *Anesthesiol Rev.* 1989; May/June: 25–9.

109. WB Pickworth, E Bunker, P Welch, E Cone. Intravenous buprenorphine reduces pupil size and the light reflex in humans. *Life Sci.* 1991; 49: 129–38.

110. O Solyman, MMI Abushanab, AR Carey, AD Henderson. Pilot study of smartphone infrared pupillography and pupillometry. *Clin Ophthalmol.* 2022; 16: 303–10.

111. C Barry, J de Souza, Y Xuan, J Holden, E Granholm. At home pupillometry using smartphone facial identification. *Proceedings of the 2022 CHI Conference on Human Factors in Computing Systems.* 2022; 235: 1–12.

112. C Barry, E Wang. Racially fair pupillometry measurements for RGB smartphone cameras using the far-red spectrum. *Sci Rep.* 2023; 13: 13841.

113. RE McKay, MA Kohn, ES Schwartz, MD Larson. Evaluation of two portable pupillometers to assess clinical utility. *Concussion.* 2020; 54: CNC82.

114. MD Larson. A new pupillometer for operating room use. *Anesthesiol Rev.* 1978; March: 41–5.

115. M Schallenberg, V Bangre, KP Steuhl, S Kremmer, JM Selbach. Comparison of the Colvard, Procyon, and Neuroptics pupillometers for measuring pupil

diameter under low ambient illumination. *J Refract Surg.* 2010; 26: 134–43.

116. SV Vellucci. The effects of ether stress and betamethasone treatment on the concentrations of norepinephrine and dopamine in various regions of the rat brain. *Br J Pharmacol.* 1977; 60: 601–5.

117. O Lowenstein, R Feinberg, IE Loewenfeld. Pupillary movements during acute and chronic fatigue. A new test for objective measurement of tiredness. *Invest Ophthal.* 1963; 2: 138–57.

118. JS Tsukahara, TL Harrison, RW Engle. The relationship between baseline pupil size and intelligence. *Cogn Psychol.* 2016; 91: 109–23.

119. M Daniel, D Charier, B Pereira, M Pachcinski, T Sharshar, S Molliex. Prognosis value of pupillometry in COVID-19 patients admitted in intensive care unit. *Auton Neurosci.* 2022; 245: 103057.

120. M Daniel, J Severinghaus, P Bickler, MD Larson. Hypoxia does not alter the human pupil diameter or the pupillary light reflex while breathing hypoxic mixtures. Anesthesiology. Abstract # 190. American Society of Anesthesiologists Annual Meeting, 1995.

121. EI McKesson. Fifty-seven years ago in anesthesia & analgesia. Nitrous oxide anesthesia: A consideration of some associated factors. *Anesth Analg.* 1932; 11: 54–9.

122. FH McMechan, L McMechan, EI McKesson. Fifty-two years ago, in anesthesia & analgesia. Elmer Isaac McKesson, MD, anesthetist: His life and work. 1937. *Anesth Analg.* 1989; 69: 259.

123. D Zhao, MH Weil, W Tang, K Klouche, SR Wann. Pupil diameter and light reaction during cardiac arrest and resuscitation. *Crit Care Med.* 2001; 2: 825–8.

124. MD Larson, AT Gray. The diagnosis of brain death. *N Engl J Med.* 2001; 345: 616–17; author reply 7–8.

125. MD Larson, J May. Effect of asphyxia on the pupils of brain-dead subjects. *Resuscitation.* 2002; 55: 31–6.

126. CL Kramer, AA Rabinstein, EF Wijdicks, SE Hocker. Neurologist versus machine: Is the pupillometer better than the naked eye in detecting pupillary reactivity? *Neurocrit Care.* 2015; 21: 309–11.

127. E Yang, M Kreuzer, S Hesse, P Davari, SC Lee, PS Garcia. Infrared pupillometry helps to detect and predict delirium in the post-anesthesia care unit. *J Clin Monit Comput.* 2018; 32: 359–68.

128. S Usui, L Stark. A model for nonlinear stochastic behavior of the pupil. *Biol Cybern.* 1982; 45: 13–21.

129. S Okamoto, M Ishizawa, S Inoue, H Sakuramoto. Use of automated infrared pupillometry to predict delirium in the intensive care unit: A prospective observational study. *SAGE Open Nurs.* 2022; 8: 23779608221124417.

130. E Favre, A Bernini, P Morelli, J Pasquier, JP Miroz, S Abed-Maillard, et al. Neuromonitoring of delirium with quantitative pupillometry in sedated mechanically ventilated critically ill patients. *Crit Care.* 2020; 24: 66.

131. S Lee, DE Jung, D Park, TJ Kim, HC Lee, J Bae, et al. Intraoperative neurological pupil index and postoperative delirium and neurologic adverse events after cardiac surgery: An observational study. *Sci Rep.* 2023; 13: 13838.

132. IE Loewenfeld, DA Newsome. Iris mechanics. I. Influence of pupil size on dynamics of pupillary movements. *Am J Ophthalmol.* 1971; 71: 347–62.

133. DA Newsome, IE Loewenfeld. Iris mechanics. II. Influence of pupil size on details of iris structure. *Am J Ophthalmol.* 1971; 71: 553–73.

134. MD Larson, A Kurz, DI Sessler, M Dechert, AR Bjorksten, F Tayefeh. Alfentanil blocks reflex pupillary dilation in response to noxious stimulation but does not diminish the

light reflex. *Anesthesiology*. 1997; 87: 849–55.

135. K Shirozu, H Setoguchi, K Tokuda, Y Karashima, M Ikeda, M Kubo, et al. The effects of anesthetic agents on pupillary function during general anesthesia using the automated infrared quantitative pupillometer. *J Clin Monit Comput*. 2017; 31: 291–6.

136. KG Belani, DI Sessler, MD Larson, MA Lopez, DE Washington, M Ozaki, et al. The pupillary light reflex. Effects of anesthetics and hyperthermia. *Anesthesiology*. 1993; 79: 23–7.

137. K Leslie, DI Sessler, WD Smith, MD Larson, M Ozaki, D Blanchard, et al. Prediction of movement during propofol/nitrous oxide anesthesia: Performance of concentration, electroencephalographic, pupillary, and hemodynamic indicators. *Anesthesiology*. 1996; 84: 52–63.

138. J Guglielminotti, F Mentre, J Gaillard, M Ghalayini, P Montravers, D Longrois. Assessment of pain during labor with pupillometry: A prospective observational study. *Anesth Analg*. 2013; 116: 1057–62.

139. RN Tyson. Simulation of cerebral death by succinylcholine sensitivity. *Arch Neurol*. 1974; 30: 409–11.

140. AT Gray, ST Krejci, MD Larson. Neuromuscular blocking drugs do not alter the pupillary light reflex of anesthetized humans. *Arch Neurol*. 1997; 54: 579–84.

141. JE Schmidt, RF Tamburro, GM Hoffman. Dilated nonreactive pupils secondary to neuromuscular blockade. *Anesthesiology*. 2000; 92: 1476–80.

142. EDP Rodrigues, GC da Costa, DQ Braga, J Pinto, MA Lessa. Rocuronium-induced dilated nonreactive pupils in a patient with coronavirus disease 2019: A case report. *A A Pract*. 2021; 15: e01491.

143. H He, Z Yu, J Zhang, W Cheng, Y Long, X Zhou, et al. Bilateral dilated nonreactive pupils secondary to rocuronium infusion in an ARDS patient treated with ECMO therapy: A case report. *Med Baltimore*. 2020; 99: e21819.

144. HM Pinheiro, RM da Costa. Pupillary light reflex as a diagnostic aid from computational viewpoint: A systematic literature review. *J Biomed Inform*. 2021; 117: 103757.

145. MD Larson, BR O'Donnell, BF Merrifield. Ocular hypothermia depresses the human pupillary light reflex. *Invest Ophthalmol Vis Sci*. 1991; 3213: 3285–7.

146. FS Southwick, PH Dalglish, Jr. Recovery after prolonged asystolic cardiac arrest in profound hypothermia. A case report and literature review. *JAMA*. 1980; 243: 1250–3.

147. KH Fischbeck, RP Simon. Neurological manifestations of accidental hypothermia. *Ann Neurol*. 1981; 10: 384–7.

148. RB Stein, T Gordon, J Shriver. Temperature dependence of mammalian muscle contractions and ATPase activities. *Biophys J*. 1982; 40: 97–107.

149. L Peluso, F Baccanelli, V Grazioli, P Panisi, FS Taccone, G Albano. Pupillary dysfunction during hypothermic circulatory arrest: Insights from automated pupillometry. *Crit Care*. 2023; 27: 197.

150. M Daniel, MD Larson, EI Eger, 2nd, M Noorani, RB Weiskopf. Fentanyl, clonidine, and repeated increases in desflurane concentration, but not nitrous oxide or esmolol, block the transient mydriasis caused by rapid increases in desflurane concentration. *Anesth Analg*. 1995; 81: 372–8.

151. RB Weiskopf, EI Eger, 2nd, M Daniel, M Noorani. Cardiovascular stimulation induced by rapid increases in desflurane concentration in humans results from activation of tracheopulmonary and systemic receptors. *Anesthesiology*. 1995; 83: 1173–8.

152. MA Moore, RB Weiskopf, EI Eger, 2nd, M Noorani, L McKay, M Damask. Rapid

1% increases of end-tidal desflurane concentration to greater than 5% transiently increase heart rate and blood pressure in humans. *Anesthesiology.* 1994; 81: 94–8.

153. MC Koss. Pupillary dilation as an index of central nervous system alpha 2 adrenergic activation. *J Pharmacol Meth.* 1986; 15: 1–19.

154. E Szabadi, C Bradshaw. Autonomic pharmacology of alpha 2 adrenoceptors. *J Psychopharmacol.* 1996; 10 Suppl. 3: 6–18.

155. S Joshi, Y Li, RM Kalwani, JI Gold. Relationships between pupil diameter and neuronal activity in the locus coeruleus, colliculi, and cingulate cortex. *Neuron.* 2016; 89: 221–34.

156. M Bonvallet, A Zbrozyna. Reticular control of the autonomic system, and particularly, the sympathetic and parasympathetic innervation of the pupil. *Arch Ital Biol.* 1963; 101: 174–207.

157. N Mullaguri, N Katyai, A Sarwai, C Newey. Pitfall in pupillometry: Exaggerated ciliospinal reflex in a patient in barbiturate coma mimicking a nonreactive pupil. *Cureus.* 2017; 9: e2004.

158. JC Andrefsky, JI Frank, D Chyatte. The ciliospinal reflex in pentobarbital coma. *J Neurosurg.* 1999; 90: 644–6.

159. EO Jørgensen, AM Malchow-Møller. Cerebral prognostic signs during cardiopulmonary resuscitation. *Resuscitation.* 1978; 64: 217–25.

160. A Reeves, J Posner. The ciliospinal response in man. *Neurology.* 1969; 19: 1145–52.

161. LL Yang, CU Niemann, MD Larson. Mechanism of pupillary reflex dilation in awake volunteers and in organ donors. *Anesthesiology.* 2003; 99: 1281–6.

162. SH Ji, SA Cho, YE Jang, EH Kim, JH Lee, JT Kim, et al. Pupil response to painful stimuli during inhalation anaesthesia without opioids in children. *Acta Anaesthesiol Scand.* 2022; 66: 803–10.

163. M Aissou, A Snauwaert, C Dupuis, A Atchabahian, F Aubrun, M Beaussier. Objective assessment of the immediate postoperative analgesia using pupillary reflex measurement: A prospective and observational study. *Anesthesiology.* 2012; 1165: 1006–12.

164. M Ossipov, G Dussor, F Porreca. Central modulation of pain. *J Clin Invest.* 2010; 120: 3779–87.

165. MD Larson, DK Gupta. Pupillary reflex dilation to predict movement: A step forward toward real-time individualized intravenous anesthetics. *Anesthesiology.* 2015; 122: 961–3.

166. J Guglielminotti, N Grillot, M Paule, F Mentre, F Servin, P Montravers, et al. Prediction of movement to surgical stimulation by the pupillary dilatation reflex amplitude evoked by a standardized noxious test. *Anesthesiology.* 2015; 122: 985–93.

167. N Marco-Arino, S Vide, M Agusti, A Chen, S Jaramillo, I Irurzun-Arana, et al. Semimechanistic models to relate noxious stimulation, movement, and pupillary dilation responses in the presence of opioids. *CPT Pharmacometrics Syst Pharmacol.* 2022; 11: 581–93.

168. HL Fields, NM Barbaro, MM Heinricher. Brain stem neuronal circuitry underlying the antinociceptive action of opiates. *Prog Brain Res.* 1988; 77: 245–57.

169. HL Fields, AI Basbaum. Brainstem control of spinal pain-transmission neurons. *Annu Rev Physiol.* 1978; 40: 217–48.

170. A Elyn, N Saffon, MD Larson. Monitoring the depth of palliative sedation by video-pupillometry: A case report. *Palliat Med.* 2021; 35: 2024–7.

171. MD Larson, PD Berry, J May, A Bjorksten, DI Sessler. Latency of pupillary reflex dilation during general anesthesia. *J Appl Physiol.* 2004; 97: 725–30.

172. MD Larson, DI Sessler, M Ozaki, J McGuire, M Schroeder. Pupillary

assessment of sensory block level during combined epidural-general anesthesia. *Anesthesiology*. 1993; 79: 42–8.

173. MD Larson, PD Berry. Supraspinal pupillary effects of intravenous and epidural fentanyl during isoflurane anesthesia. *Reg Anesth Pain Med*. 2000; 25: 60–6.

174. S Isnardon, M Vinclair, C Genty, A Hebrard, P Albaladejo, JF Payen. Pupillometry to detect pain response during general anaesthesia following unilateral popliteal sciatic nerve block: A prospective, observational study. *Eur J Anaesthesiol*. 2013; 30: 429–34.

175. MD Larson, RS Fung, AJ Infosino, A Baba. Efficacy of epidural block during general anesthesia. *Anesthesiology*. 2006; 105: 632–3.

176. A Migeon, FP Desgranges, D Chassard, BJ Blaise, et al. Pupillary reflex dilation and analgesia nociception index monitoring to assess the effectiveness of regional anesthesia in children anesthetised with sevoflurane. *Pediatr Anesth*. 2013. 23: 1160–5.

177. L Barvais, E Engelman, JM Eba, E Coussaert, F Cantraine, GN Kenny. Effect site concentrations of remifentanil and pupil response to noxious stimulation. *Br J Anaesth*. 2003; 91: 347–52.

178. I Constant, MC Nghe, L Boudet, J Berniere, S Schrayer, R Seeman, et al. Reflex pupillary dilatation in response to skin incision and alfentanil in children anaesthetized with sevoflurane: A more sensitive measure of noxious stimulation than the commonly used variables. *Br J Anaesth*. 2006; 96: 614–19.

179 D Ly-Liu, F Reinoso-Barbero. Immediate postoperative pain can also be predicted by pupillary pain index in children. *Br J Anaesth*. 2015; 114: 345–6.

180. N Sabourdin, L Del Bove, N Louvet, S Luzon-Chetrit, B Tavernier, I Constant. Relationship between pre-incision Pupillary Pain Index and post-incision heart rate and pupillary diameter variation in children. *Paediatr Anaesth*. 2021; 31: 1121–8.

181. M Vinclair, C Schilte, F Roudaud, J Lavolaine, G Francony, P Bouzat, et al. Using Pupillary Pain Index to assess nociception in sedated critically ill patients. *Anesth Analg*. 2019; 129: 1540–6.

182. E Macchini, A Bertelli, EG Bogossian, F Annoni, A Minini, A Quispe Cornejo, et al. Pain pupillary index to prognosticate unfavorable outcome in comatose cardiac arrest patients. *Resuscitation*. 2022; 176: 125–31.

183. D Charier, M Vogler, D Zantor, V Pichot, A Baltar, M Courbon, et al. Assessing pain in the postoperative period: Analgesia nociception index vs pupillometry. *Brit J Anaesth*. 2019; 123: 322–7.

184. DJ Charier, D Zantour, V Pichot, F Chouchou, JM Barthelemy, F Roche, et al. Assessing pain using the variation coefficient of pupillary diameter. *J Pain*. 2017; 18: 1346–53.

185. C Gregoire, D Charier, R de Bergeyck, A Mouraux, F Van Ouytsel, R Lambert, et al. Comparison between pupillometry and numeric pain rating scale for pain assessments in communicating adult patients in the emergency department. *Eur J Pain*. 2023; 27: 952–60.

186. TJ Lynch, R Siminoff, R Podolsky, MW Adler. Morphine-induced pupillary fluctuations in the rat: Correlations with EEG and respiratory changes. *J Ocul Pharmacol*. 1985; 1: 255–61.

187. RB Murray, MW Adler, AD Korczyn. The pupillary effects of opioids. *Life Sci*. 1983; 33: 495–509.

188. MP Bokoch, M Behrends, A Neice, MD Larson. Fentanyl, an agonist at the mu opioid receptor, depresses pupillary unrest. *Auton Neurosci*. 2015; 189: 68–74.

189. A Neice, T Ma, K Chang. Relationship between age, sex and pupillary unrest. *J Clin Monit Comput*. 2022; 36: 1897–901.

190. L Stark. Stability, oscillations, and noise in the human pupil servomechanism. *Bol Inst Estud Med Biol Univ Nac Auton Mex.* 1963; 21: 201–22.

191. P Turnbull, N Irani, N Lim, J Phillips. Origins of pupillary hippus in the autonomic nervous system. *Invest Ophthalmol Vis Sci.* 2017; 58: 197–203.

192. B Wilhelm, H Wilhelm, H Ludtke, P Streicher, M Adler. Pupillographic assessment of sleepiness in sleep-deprived healthy subjects. *Sleep.* 1998; 21: 258–65.

193. B Wilhelm, H Giedke, H Ludtke, E Bittner, A Hofmann, H Wilhelm. Daytime variations in central nervous system activation measured by a pupillographic sleepiness test. *J Sleep Res.* 2001; 10: 1–7.

194. B Wilhelm, R Kellert, R Schnell, H Ludtke, O Petrini. Lack of sedative effects after vespertine intake of oxazepam as hypnotic in healthy volunteers. *Psychopharmacol Berl.* 2009; 205: 679–88.

195. B Wilhelm, G Stuiber, H Ludtke, H Wilhelm. The effect of caffeine on spontaneous pupillary oscillations. *Ophthalmic Physiol Opt.* 2014; 34: 73–81.

196. BJ Wilhelm, A Widmann, W Durst, C Heine, G Otto. Objective and quantitative analysis of daytime sleepiness in physicians after night duties. *Int J Psychophysiol.* 2009; 72: 307–13.

197. G Aston-Jones, JD Cohen. An integrative theory of locus coeruleus-norepinephrine function: Adaptive gain and optimal performance. *Annu Rev Neurosci.* 2005; 28: 403–50.

198. MS Gilzenrat, S Nieuwenhuis, M Jepma, JD Cohen. Pupil diameter tracks changes in control state predicted by the adaptive gain theory of locus coeruleus function. *Cogn Affect Behav Neurosci.* 2010; 10: 252–69.

199. A Pome, DC Burr, A Capuozzo, P Binda. Spontaneous pupillary oscillations increase during mindfulness meditation. *Curr Biol.* 2020; 30: R1030–R1031.

200. R Rubin, LF Abbott, H Sompolinsky. Balanced excitation and inhibition are required for high-capacity, noise-robust neuronal selectivity. *Proc Natl Acad Sci USA.* 2017; 114: E9366–E9375.

201. MD Larson. Effect of ambient light on pupillary reflex dilation during general anesthesia. 26th Pupil Colloquium, Bear Mountain, New York. 2005.

202. M Steriade. *The Intact and Sliced Brain.* Cambridge, MA: MIT Press; 2001.

203. M Devor, V Zalkind, Y Fishman, A Minert. Model of anaesthetic induction by unilateral intracerebral microinjection of GABAergic agonists. *Eur J Neurosci.* 2016; 43: 846–58.

204. E Szabadi. Modulation of physiological reflexes by pain: Role of the locus coeruleus. *Front Integr Neurosci.* 2012; 6: 94.

205. M Megemont, J McBurney-Lin, H Yang. Pupil diameter is not an accurate real-time readout of locus coeruleus activity. *Elife.* 2022; 11: E70510.

206. Y Yu, MC Koss. Alpha2-adrenoceptors do not mediate reflex mydriasis in rabbits. *J Ocul Pharmacol Ther.* 2004; 20: 479–88.

207. WB Pickworth, LG Sharpe. Morphine-induced mydriasis and inhibition of pupillary light reflex and fluctuations in the cat. *J Pharmacol Exp Ther.* 1985; 234: 603–6.

208. LG Sharpe, WB Pickworth. Pharmacologic evidence for a tonic muscarinic inhibitory input to the Edinger-Westphal nucleus in the dog. *Exp Neurol.* 1981; 711: 176–90.

209. FF Weight, GC Salmoiraghi. Responses of spinal cord interneurons to acetylcholine, norepinephrine, and serotonin administered by microelectrophoresis. *J Pharmacol Exp Ther.* 1966; 1533: 420–7.

210. C Batini, G Moruzzi, M Palestini, GF Rossi, A Zanchetti. Presistent patterns of wakefulness in the pretrigeminal midpontine preparation. *Science.* 1958; 128: 30–2.

211. T Yoshitomi, Y Ito. Double reciprocal innervations in dog iris sphincter and dilator muscles. *Invest Ophthalmol Vis Sci.* 1986; 27: 83–91.

212. T Yoshitomi, Y Ito, H Inomata. Adrenergic excitatory and cholinergic inhibitory innervations in the human iris dilator. *Exp Eye Res.* 1985; 40: 453–9.

213. LA Santa Cruz Mercado, R Liu, KM Bharadwaj, JJ Johnson, R Gutierrez, P Das, et al. Association of intraoperative opioid administration with postoperative pain and opioid use. *JAMA Surg.* 2023; 158: 854–64.

214. N Sabourdin, J Barrois, N Louvet, A Rigouzzo, ML Guye, C Dadure, et al. Pupillometry-guided intraoperative remifentanil administration versus standard practice influences opioid use: A randomized study. *Anesthesiology.* 2017; 127: 284–92.

215. MD Larson. Mechanism of opioid-induced pupillary effects. *Clin Neurophysiol.* 2008; 119: 1358–64.

216. G Berlucchi, G Morruzzi, G Salvi, P Strata. Pupil behavior and ocular movements during synchronized and desynchronized sleep. *Arch Ital Biol.* 1964; 102: 230–44.

217. N Ichinohe, K Shoumura. Marked miosis caused by deafferenting the oculomotor nuclear complex in the cat. *Auton Neurosci.* 2001; 94: 42–5.

218. CW Vaughan, MJ Christie. Presynaptic inhibitory action of opioids on synaptic transmission in the rat periaqueductal grey in vitro. *J Physiol.* 1997; 498 Pt 2: 463–72.

219. DA Newsome. Afterimage and pupillary activity following strong light exposure. *Vision Res.* 1971; 11: 275–88.

220. M Behrends, MD Larson, A Neice, M Bokoch. Suppression of pupillary unrest by general anesthesia and propofol sedation. *J Clin Monit Comput.* 2018; 332: 317–23.

221. G Teasdale, B Jennett. Assessment of coma and impaired consciousness: A practical scale. *Lancet.* 1974; 2: 81–4.

222. EF Wijdicks, WR Bamlet, BV Maramattom, EM Manno, RL McClelland. Validation of a new coma scale: The FOUR score. *Ann Neurol.* 2005; 58: 585–93.

223. PM Brennan, GD Murray, GM Teasdale. Simplifying the use of prognostic information in traumatic brain injury. Part 1: The GCS-Pupils score: An extended index of clinical severity. *J Neurosurg.* 2018; 128: 1612–20.

224. E Dowlati, K Sarpong, S Kamande, AH Carroll, J Murray, A Wiley, et al. Abnormal neurological pupil index is associated with malignant cerebral edema after mechanical thrombectomy in large vessel occlusion patients. *Neurol Sci.* 2021; 42: 5139–48.

225. M Bower, A Sweidan, J Xu, S Stern-Neze, W Yu, L Groysman. Quantitative pupillometry in the intensive care unit. *J Intensive Care Med.* 2021; 36: 383–91.

226. WR Taylor, JW Chen, H Meltzer, TA Gennarelli, C Kelbch, S Knowlton, et al. Quantitative pupillometry, a new technology: Normative data and preliminary observations in patients with acute head injury: Technical note. *J Neurosurg.* 2003; 98: 205–13.

227. SF Zafar, JI Suarez. Automated pupillometer for monitoring the critically ill patient: A critical appraisal. *J Crit Care.* 2014; 29: 599–603.

228. BL Lussier, M Erapuram, JA White, SE Stutzman, DM Olson. Predictive value of quantitative pupillometry in patients with normal pressure hydrocephalus undergoing temporary CSF diversion. *Neurol Sci.* 2022; 43: 5377–82.

229. BL Lussier, DM Olson, V Aiyagari. Automated pupillometry in neurocritical care: Research and practice. *Curr Neurol Neurosci Rep.* 2019; 19: 71.

230. M Osman, SE Stutzman, F Atem, D Olson, AD Hicks, S Ortega-Perez, et al. Correlation of objective pupillometry to midline shift in acute

stroke patients. *J Stroke Cerebrovasc Dis.* 2019; 28: 1902–10.

231. TJ Kim, SB Ko. Implication of neurological pupil index for monitoring of brain edema. *Acute Crit Care.* 2018; 33: 57–60.

232. S Packiasabapathy, V Rangasamy, S Sadhasivam. Pupillometry in perioperative medicine: A narrative review. *Can J Anaesth.* 2021; 68: 566–78.

233. JW Chen, ZJ Gombart, S Rogers, SK Gardiner, S Cecil, RM Bullock. Pupillary reactivity as an early indicator of increased intracranial pressure: The introduction of the neurological pupil index. *Surg Neurol Int.* 2011; 2: 82.

234. DM Olson, M Fishel. The use of automated pupillometry in critical care. *Crit Care Nurs Clin North Am.* 2016; 28: 101–7.

235. C Sandroni, F Cavallaro, CW Callaway, S D'Arrigo, T Sanna, MA Kuiper, et al. Predictors of poor neurological outcome in adult comatose survivors of cardiac arrest: A systematic review and meta-analysis. Part 2: Patients treated with therapeutic hypothermia. *Resuscitation.* 2015; 84: 1324–38.

236. C Sandroni, JP Nolan, LW Andersen, BW Bottiger, A Cariou, T Cronberg, et al. ERC-ESICM guidelines on temperature control after cardiac arrest in adults. *Intensive Care Med.* 2022; 48: 261–9.

237. T Suys, P Bouzat, P Marques-Vidal, N Sala, JF Payen, AO Rossetti, et al. Automated quantitative pupillometry for the prognostication of coma after cardiac arrest. *Neurocrit Care.* 2014; 21: 300–8.

238. RR Riker, ME Sawyer, VG Fischman, T May, C Lord, A Eldridge, et al. Neurological pupil index and pupillary light reflex by pupillometry predict outcome early after cardiac arrest. *Neurocrit Care.* 2020; 32: 152–61.

239. T Tamura, J Namiki, Y Sugawara, K Sekine, K Yo, T Kanaya, et al. Early outcome prediction with quantitative pupillary response parameters after out-of-hospital cardiac arrest: A multicenter prospective observational study. *PLoS One.* 2020; 15: e0228224.

240. T Tamura, J Namiki, Y Sugawara, K Sekine, K Yo, T Kanaya, et al. Quantitative assessment of pupillary light reflex for early prediction of outcomes after out-of-hospital cardiac arrest: A multicentre prospective observational study. *Resuscitation.* 2018; 131: 108–13.

241. M Oddo, C Sandroni, G Citerio, JP Miroz, J Horn, M Rundgren, et al. Quantitative versus standard pupillary light reflex for early prognostication in comatose cardiac arrest patients: An international prospective multicenter double-blinded study. *Intensive Care Med.* 2018; 44: 2102–11.

242. J Godau, K Bharad, J Rosche, G Nagy, S Kastner, K Weber, et al. Automated pupillometry for assessment of treatment success in nonconvulsive status epilepticus. *Neurocrit Care.* 2022; 36: 148–56.

243. S Yan, Z Tu, W Lu, Q Zhang, J He, Z Li, et al. Clinical utility of an automated pupillometer for assessing and monitoring recipients of liver transplantation. *Liver Transpl.* 2009; 15: 1718–27.

244. JP Miroz, N Ben-Hamouda, A Bernini, F Romagnosi, F Bongiovanni, A Roumy, et al. Neurological pupil index for early prognostication after venoarterial extracorporeal membrane oxygenation. *Chest.* 2020; 157: 1167–74.

245. H Lee, SH Choi, B Park, YH Hong, HB Lee, SB Jeon. Quantitative assessments of pupillary light reflexes in hospital-onset unresponsiveness. *BMC Neurol.* 2021; 21: 234.

246. C Ong, M Hutch, M Barra, A Kim, S Zafar, S Smirnakis. Effects of osmotic therapy on pupil reactivity: Quantification using pupillometry in critically ill neurologic patients. *Neurocrit Care.* 2019; 30: 307–15.

247. L Peluso, L Ferlini, M Talamonti, N Ndieugnou Djangang, E Gouvea

Bogossian, M Menozzi, et al. Automated pupillometry for prediction of electroencephalographic reactivity in critically ill patients: A prospective cohort study. *Front Neurol.* 2022; 13: 867603.

248. L Peluso, M Oddo, C Sandroni, G Citerio, FS Taccone. Early neurological pupil index to predict outcome after cardiac arrest. *Intensive Care Med.* 2022; 48: 496–7.

249. J Hutchinson. Notes on the symptom – significance of different states of the pupil. *Brain.* 1878; 1: 1–13.

250. AH Ropper. The opposite pupil in herniation. *Neurology.* 1990; 40: 1707–9.

251. GT Manley, MD Larson. Infrared pupillometry during uncal herniation. *J Neurosurg Anesthesiol.* 2002; 14: 223–8.

252. TY El Ahmadieh, N Bedros, SE Stutzman, D Nyancho, AM Venkatachalam, M MacAllister, et al. Automated pupillometry as a triage and assessment tool in patients with traumatic brain injury. *World Neurosurg.* 2021; 145: e163–e169.

253. JI Traylor, TY El Ahmadieh, NM Bedros, N Al Adli, SE Stutzman, AM Venkatachalam, et al. Quantitative pupillometry in patients with traumatic brain injury and loss of consciousness: A prospective pilot study. *J Clin Neurosci.* 2021; 91: 88–92.

254. KJ Ciuffreda, NR Joshi, JQ Truong. Understanding the effects of mild traumatic brain injury on the pupillary light reflex. *Concussion.* 2017; 2: CNC36.

255. A Helmy, PJ Kirkpatrick, HM Seeley, E Corteen, DK Menon, PJ Hutchinson. Fixed, dilated pupils following traumatic brain injury: Historical perspectives, causes and ophthalmological sequelae. *Acta Neurochir Suppl.* 2012; 114: 295–9.

256. JQ Truong, KJ Ciuffreda. Comparison of pupillary dynamics to light in the mild traumatic brain injury (mTBI) and normal populations. *Brain Inj.* 2016; 30: 1378–89.

257. JQ Truong, KJ Ciuffreda. Quantifying pupillary asymmetry through objective binocular pupillometry in the normal and mild traumatic brain injury (mTBI) populations. *Brain Inj.* 2016; 30: 1372–7.

258. A Condemi, G Donatiello, M Mauro, A Spazzolini, C Zocchi. Importance of pupillary and photomotor reflexes in cardiac resuscitation. *Minerva Anestesiol.* 1981; 47: 885–90.

259. H Obinata, S Yokobori, Y Shibata, T Takiguchi, R Nakae, Y Igarashi, et al. Early automated infrared pupillometry is superior to auditory brainstem response in predicting neurological outcome after cardiac arrest. *Resuscitation.* 2020; 154: 77–84.

260. J Pansell, R Hack, P Rudberg, M Bell, C Cooray. Can quantitative pupillometry be used to screen for elevated intracranial pressure? A retrospective cohort study. *Neurocrit Care.* 2022; 37: 531–7.

261. S Paramanathan, AM Grejs, E Soreide, CHV Duez, AN Jeppesen, AJ Reinertsen, et al. Quantitative pupillometry in comatose out-of-hospital cardiac arrest patients: A post-hoc analysis of the TTH48 trial. *Acta Anaesthesiol Scand.* 2022; 66: 880–6.

262. L Shi, J Xu, J Wang, M Zhang, F Liu, ZU Khan, et al. Automated pupillometry helps monitor the efficacy of cardiopulmonary resuscitation and predict return of spontaneous circulation. *Am J Emerg Med.* 2021; 49: 360–6.

263. A Warren, C McCarthy, M Andiapen, M Crouch, S Finney, S Hamilton, et al. Early quantitative infrared pupillometry for prediction of neurological outcome in patients admitted to intensive care after out-of-hospital cardiac arrest. *Br J Anaesth.* 2022; 128: 849–56.

264. N Ben-Hamouda, Z Ltaief, M Kirsch, J Novy, L Liaudet, M Oddo, et al. Neuroprognostication under ECMO after cardiac arrest: Are classical tools still performant? *Neurocrit Care.* 2022; 37: 293–301.

265. B Nyholm, LER Obling, C Hassager, J Grand, JE Moller, MH Othman, et al.

Specific thresholds of quantitative pupillometry parameters predict unfavorable outcome in comatose survivors early after cardiac arrest. *Resusc Plus.* 2023; 14: 100399.

266. PD Levy, H Ye, S Compton, PS Chan, GL Larkin, RD Welch. Factors associated with neurologically intact survival for patients with acute heart failure and in-hospital cardiac arrest. *Circ Heart Fail.* 2009; 2: 572–81.

267. WT Longstreth, Jr., P Diehr, TS Inui, EO Jorgensen, AM Malchow-Moller. Prediction of awakening after out-of-hospital cardiac arrest. *N Engl J Med.* 1983; 308: 1378–82.

268. MG Goetting, E Contreras. Systemic atropine administration during cardiac arrest does not cause fixed and dilated pupils. *Ann Emerg Med.* 1991; 20: 55–7.

269. V Rajajee, S Muehlschlegel, KE Wartenberg, SA Alexander, KM Busl, SHY Chou, et al. Guidelines for neuroprognostication in comatose adult survivors of cardiac arrest. *Neurocrit Care.* 2023; 38: 533–63.

270. AR Panchal, JA Bartos, JG Cabanas, MW Donnino, IR Drennan, KG Hirsch, et al. Part 3: Adult basic and advanced life support: 2020 American Heart Association guidelines for cardiopulmonary resuscitation and emergency cardiovascular care. *Circulation.* 2020; 142: S366–S468.

271. A Monk, S Patil. Infrared pupillometry to help predict neurological outcome for patients achieving return of spontataneous circulation following cardiac arrest: A systematic review protocol. *Syst Rev.* 2019; 8: 286. Published online.

272. M Menozzi, M Oddo, L Peluso, G Dessartaine, C Sandroni, G Citerio, et al. Early neurological pupil index assessment to predict outcome in cardiac arrest patients undergoing extracorporeal membrane oxygenation. *ASAIO J.* 2022; 68: e118–e120.

273. D Kondziella. Neuroprognostication after cardiac arrest: What the cardiologist should know. *Eur Heart J Acute Cardiovasc Care.* 2023; 12: 550–8.

274. AO Rossetti, AA Rabinstein, M Oddo. Neurological prognostication of outcome in patients in coma after cardiac arrest. *Lancet Neurol.* 2016; 15: 597–609.

275. JC Slovis, A Bach, F Beaulieu, G Zuckerberg, A Topjian, MP Kirschen. Neuromonitoring after pediatric cardiac arrest: Cerebral physiology and injury stratification. *Neurocrit Care.* 2024; 40: 99–115.

276. KM Berg, A Cheng, AR Panchal, AA Topjian, K Aziz, F Bhanji, et al. Part 7: Systems of care: 2020 American Heart Association guidelines for cardiopulmonary resuscitation and emergency cardiovascular care. *Circulation.* 2020; 14216 Suppl. 2: S580–S604.

277. PF Binnion, RJ McFarland. The relationship between cardiac massage and pupil size in cardiac arrest in dogs. *Cardiovasc Res.* 1968; 23: 247–51.

278. P Sobotka, E Gebert. Effect of complete brain ischaemia on pupillary changes. *Acta Anaesthesiol Scand.* 1972; 16: 112–16.

279. JE Steen-Hansen, NN Hansen, P Vaagenes, B Schreiner, WT Longstreth, Jr., P Diehr, et al. Pupil size and light reactivity during cardiopulmonary resuscitation: A clinical study. *Crit Care Med.* 1988; 16: 69–70.

280. DW Kim, YH Jo, SM Park, DK Lee, D Jang. Neurological pupil index during cardiopulmonmary resuscitation is associated with admission to ICU in non-traumatic out-of-hospital cardiac arrest patients. *Signa Vitae.* 2023; 19: 48–54.

281. RM Merchant, AA Topjian, AR Panchal, A Cheng, K Aziz, KM Berg, et al. Part 1: Executive summary: 2020 American Heart Association guidelines for cardiopulmonary resuscitation and emergency cardiovascular care. *Circulation.* 2020; 142 Suppl. 2: S337–S357.

282. M Behrends, CU Niemann, MD Larson. Infrared pupillometry to detect the light reflex during cardiopulmonary resuscitation: A case series. *Resuscitation.* 2012; 83: 1223–8.

283. FD Bremner, SE Smith. Bilateral tonic pupils: Holmes Adie syndrome or generalized neuropathy? *Br J Ophthalmol.* 2007; 91: 1620–3.

284. JL Ang, S Collis, B Dhillon, P Cackett. The eye in forensic medicine: A narrative review. *Asia Pac J Ophthalmol Phila.* 2021; 10: 486–94.

285. G Olgun, CR Newey, A Ardelt. Pupillometry in brain death: Differences in pupillary diameter between paediatric and adult subjects. *Neurol Res.* 2015; 37: 945–50.

286. D Kondziella, A Bender, K Diserens, W van Erp, A Estraneo, R Formisano, et al. European Academy of Neurology guideline on the diagnosis of coma and other disorders of consciousness. *Eur J Neurol.* 2020; 275: 741–56.

287. A Vassilieva, MH Olsen, C Peinkhofer, GM Knudsen, D Kondziella. Automated pupillometry to detect command following in neurological patients: A proof-of-concept study. *PeerJ.* 2019; 7: e6929.

288. EW Jakobsen, V Nersesjan, SS Albrechtsen, MH Othman, M Amiri, NV Knudsen, et al. Brimonidine eye drops reveal diminished sympathetic pupillary tone in comatose patients with brain injury. *Acta Neurochir (Wien).* 2023; 165: 1483–94.

289. LG Sharpe, WB Pickworth. Opposite pupillary size effects in the cat and dog after microinjections of morphine, normorphine and clonidine in the Edinger-Westphal nucleus. *Brain Res Bull.* 1985; 15: 329–33.

290. MD Rollins, JR Feiner, JM Lee, S Shah, M Larson. Pupillary effects of high-dose opioid quantified with infrared pupillometry. *Anesthesiology.* 2014; 121: 1037–44.

291. IE Loewenfeld. The iris as pharmacologic indicator. I. Effect of physostigmine and of pilocarpine on pupillary movements in normal man. *Arch Ophthalmol.* 1963; 70: 42–51.

292. L Weinhold, G Bigelow. Opioid miosis: Effects of lighting intensity and monocular and binocular exposure. *Drug Alcohol Depend.* 1993; 31: 177–81.

293. LL Weinhold, GE Bigelow. Factors influencing assessment of opioid miosis in humans. *NIDA Res Monogr.* 1990; 105: 419–20.

294. JH Pula, AM Kao, JC Kattah. Neuro-ophthalmologic side-effects of systemic medications. *Curr Opin Ophthalmol.* 2013; 24: 540–9.

295. K Pattinson. Opioids and the control of respiration. *Br J Anaesth.* 2008; 100: 747–58.

296. ED Kharasch, A Francis, A London, K Frey, T Kim, J Blood. Sensitivity of intravenous and oral alfentanil and pupillary miosis as minimal and noninvasive probes for hepatic and first-pass CYP3A induction. *Clin Pharmacol Ther.* 2005; 90: 100–8.

297. ED Kharasch, C Hoffer, A Walker, P Sheffels. Disposition and miotic effects of oral alfentanil: A potential noninvasive probe for first-pass cytochrome P4503A activity. *Clin Pharmacol Ther.* 2003; 73: 199–208.

298. ED Kharasch, C Hoffer, D Whittington. Influence of age on the pharmacokinetics and pharmacodynamics of oral transmucosal fentanyl citrate. *Anesthesiology.* 2004; 101: 738–43.

299. ED Kharasch, C Hoffer, D Whittington, P Sheffels. Role of P-glycoprotein in the intestinal absorption and clinical effects of morphine. *Clin Pharmacol Ther.* 2003; 74: 543–54.

300. ED Kharasch, A Walker, C Hoffer, P Sheffels. Intravenous and oral alfentanil as in vivo probes for hepatic and first-pass cytochrome P450 3A activity: Noninvasive assessment by use of pupillary miosis. *Clin Pharmacol Ther.* 2004; 76: 452–66.

301. ED Kharasch, A Walker, C Hoffer, P Sheffels. Sensitivity of intravenous and oral alfentanil and pupillary miosis as minimally invasive and noninvasive probes for hepatic and first-pass CYP3A activity. *J Clin Pharmacol.* 2005; 45: 1187–97.

302. AH Ghodse, TH Bewley, MK Kearney, SE Smith. Mydriatic response to topical naloxone in opiate abusers. *Br J Psychiatry.* 1986; 148: 44–6.

303. MD Larson. Action of narcotics on the pupil. *Anaesthesia.* 1987; 42: 566.

304. AW Duggan, RA North. Electrophysiology of opioids. *Pharmacol Rev.* 1983; 35: 219–81.

305. J Semmlow, D Hansmann, L Stark. Variation in pupillomotor responsiveness with mean pupil size. *Vision Res.* 1975; 15: 85–90.

306. JP Kollars, MD Larson. Tolerance to miotic effects of opioids. *Anesthesiology.* 2005; 1023: 701.

307. L Lee, R Caplan, L Stephens, K Posner, G Terman, T Voepel-Lewis, et al. Postoperative opioid-induced respiratory depression: A closed claims analysis. *Anesthesiology.* 2015; 122: 659–65.

308. V Solhaug, E Molden. Individual variability in clinical effect and tolerability of opioid analgesics: Importance of drug interactions and pharmacogenetics. *Scand J Pain.* 2017; 17: 193–200.

309. R Du, M Meeker, P Bacchetti, MD Larson, MC Holland, GT Manley. Evaluation of the portable infrared pupillometer. *Neurosurgery.* 2005; 57: 198–203.

310. RE McKay, MD Larson. Detection of opioid effect with pupillometry. *Auton Neurosci.* 2021; 235: 102869.

311. CW Vaughan, SL Ingram, MA Connor, MJ Christie. How opioids inhibit GABA-mediated neurotransmission. *Nature.* 1997; 390: 611–14.

312. GK Aghajanian, YY Wang. Common alpha 2- and opiate effector mechanisms in the locus coeruleus: Intracellular studies in brain slices. *Neuropharmacology.* 1987; 26: 793–9.

313. RE McKay, AE Neice, MD Larson. Pupillary unrest in ambient light and prediction of opioid responsiveness: Case report on its utility in the management of 2 patients with challenging acute pain conditions. *A A Pract.* 2018; 1010: 279–82.

314. J Lundy. *Clinical Anesthesia: A Manual of Clinical Anesthesiology.* Philadelphia, PA: W. B. Saunders; 1942.

315. RE McKay, MA Kohn, MD Larson. Pupillary unrest, opioid intensity, and the impact of environmental stimulation on respiratory depression. *J Clin Monit Comput.* 2022; 36: 473–82.

316. F Borghjerg, K Nielsen, J Franks. Experimental pain stimulates respiration and attenuates morphine-induced respiratory depression: A controlled study in human volunteers. *Pain.* 1996; 64: 123–8.

317. AE Neice, M Behrends, MP Bokoch, KM Seligman, NM Conrad, MD Larson. Prediction of opioid analgesic efficacy by measurement of pupillary unrest. *Anesth Analg.* 2017; 124: 915–21.

318. JD Smith, LY Ichinose, GA Masek, T Watanabe, L Stark. Midbrain single units correlating with pupil response to light. *Science.* 1968; 162: 1302–3.

319. M Behrends, MD Larson. Measurements of pupillary unrest using infrared pupillometry fail to detect changes in pain intensity in patients after surgery: A prospective observational study. *Can J Anesth.* 2024; published online ahead of print: https://pubmed.ncbi.nlm.nih.gov/38504035/

320. J Eisenach, R Curry, C Aschenbrenner, R Coghill, T Houle. Pupil responses and pain ratings to heat stimuli: Reliability and effects of expectations and a conditioning pain stimulus. *J Neurosci Methods.* 2017; 279: 52–9.

321. SE Smith, SA Smith, PM Brown, C Fox, PH Sonksen. Pupillary signs in diabetic

autonomic neuropathy. *Brit Med J.* 1978; 2: 924–7.

322. PF Kaeser, A Kawasaki. Disorders of pupillary structure and function. *Neurol Clin.* 28: 657–77.

323. HS Thompson, SF Piley. Unequal pupils. A flow chart for sorting out the anisocorias. *Surv Ophthalmol.* 1976; 21: 45–8.

324. JS Czarnecki, SF Pilley, HS Thompson. The analysis of anisocoria. The use of photography in the clinical evaluation of unequal pupils. *Can J Ophthalmol.* 1979; 14: 297–302.

325. AA Antonio-Santos, RN Santo, ER Eggenberger. Pharmacological testing of anisocoria. *Expert Opin Pharmacother.* 2005; 6: 2007–13.

326. JA Stirt, JR Shuptrine, CS Sternick, GA Korbon. Anisocoria after anaesthesia. *Can Anaesth Soc J.* 1985; 32: 422–4.

327. RC Prielipp. Unilateral mydriasis after induction of anaesthesia. *Can J Anaesth.* 1994; 41: 140–3.

328. MM Rubin, RS Sadoff, GM Cozzi. Postoperative unilateral mydriasis due to phenylephrine: A case report. *J Oral Maxillofac Surg.* 1990; 48: 621–3.

329. BT Sitzman, DL Bogdonoff, TP Bleck, BF Spiekermann, CW Chang. Postoperative anisocoria: Neurogenic or phenylephrine induced? A rapid diagnostic test. *Anesth Analg.* 1996; 83: 633–5.

330. YC Lin. Anisocoria from transdermal scopolamine. *Paediatr Anaesth.* 2001; 11: 626–7.

331. SN Al-Holou, SN Lipsky, BN Wasserman. Don't sweat the blown pupil: Anisocoria in patients using qbrexza. *Ophthalmology.* 2020; 127: 1381.

332. WC Holmgreen, HM Baddour, HB Tilson. Unilateral mydriasis during general anesthesia. *J Oral Surg.* 1979; 37: 740–2.

333. MG D'Souza, A Hadzic, T Wider. Unilateral mydriasis after nasal reconstruction surgery. *Can J Anaesth.* 2000; 47: 1119–21.

334. BE Gibson, RJ Stanley, WL Lanier. Prolonged unilateral mydriasis after nasal septal reconstruction. *Anesth Analg.* 1987; 66: 197–8.

335. M Jindal, N Sharma, N Parekh. Intraoperative dilated pupil during nasal polypectomy. *Eur Arch Otorhinolaryngol.* 2009; 266: 1035–7.

336. MT Bhatti. Neuro-ophthalmic complications of endoscopic sinus surgery. *Curr Opin Ophthalmol.* 2007; 18: 450–8.

337. MT Bhatti, JA Stankiewicz. Ophthalmic complications of endoscopic sinus surgery. *Surv Ophthalmol.* 2003; 48: 389–402.

338. SG Boynes, Z Echeverria, M Abdulwahab. Ocular complications associated with local anesthesia administration in dentistry. *Dent Clin North Am.* 54: 677–86.

339. J Horowitz, Y Almog, A Wolf, G Buckman, O Geyer. Ophthalmic complications of dental anesthesia: Three new cases. *J Neuroophthalmol.* 2005; 25: 95–100.

340. M Penarrocha-Diago, JM Sanchis-Bielsa. Ophthalmologic complications after intraoral local anesthesia with articaine. *Oral Surg Oral Med Oral Pathol Oral Radiol Endod.* 2000; 90: 21–4.

341. JD Mason, RJ Haynes, NS Jones. Interpretation of the dilated pupil during endoscopic sinus surgery. *J Laryngol Otol.* 1998; 112: 622–7.

342. SW Hyams. Oculomotor palsy following dental anesthesia. *Arch Ophthalmol.* 1976; 94: 1281–2.

343. C Rene, GE Rose, R Lenthall, I Moseley. Major orbital complications of endoscopic sinus surgery. *Br J Ophthalmol.* 2001; 85: 598–603.

344. S Rayatt, A Khanna. Unilateral mydriasis during blepharoplasty. *Br J Plast Surg.* 2001; 54: 648.

345. JP Perlman, H Conn. Transient internal ophthalmoplegia during blepharoplasty.

A report of three cases. *Ophthal Plast Reconstr Surg.* 1991; 7: 141–3.

346. F Bremner. Pupil evaluation as a test for autonomic disorders. *Clin Auton Res.* 2009; 192: 88–101.

347. JA Emelifeonwu, K Reid, JK Rhodes, L Myles. Saved by the pupillometer! – A role for pupillometry in the acute assessment of patients with traumatic brain injuries? *Brain Inj.* 2018; 32: 675–7.

348. MD Larson, I Muhiudeen. Pupillometric analysis of the "absent light reflex." *Arch Neurol.* 1995; 52: 369–72.

349. MB Maas, AM Naidech, A Batra, SH Chou, TP Bleck. Comment on "Can quantitative pupillometry be used to screen for elevated intracranial pressure"? A retrospective cohort study. *Neurocrit Care.* 2022; 37: 597–8.

350. B Nyholm, L Obling, C Hassager, J Grand, J Moller, M Othman, et al. Superior reproducibility, and repeatability in automated quantitative pupillometry compared to standard manual assessment, and quantitative pupillary response parameters present high reliability in critically ill cardiac patients. *PLoS One.* 2022; 17: e0272303.

351. A Blandino Ortiz, J Higuera Lucas. Usefulness of quantitative pupillometry in the intensive care unit. *Med Intensiva England.* 2022; 46: 273–6.

352. A Blandino Ortiz, J Higuera Lucas, C Soriano, R de Pablo. Quantitative pupillometry as a tool to predict post-cardiac arrest neurological outcome in target temperature patients. *Med Intensiva England.* 2022; 4: 415.

353. D Bouyaknouden, TN Peddada, N Ravishankar, S Fatima, J Fong-Isariyawongse, EJ Gilmore, et al. Neurological prognostication after hypoglycemic coma: Role of clinical and EEG findings. *Neurocrit Care.* 2022; 37: 273–80.

354. YA Campos, P Rana, RG Reyes, K Mazhar, SE Stutzman, F Atem, et al. Relationship between automated pupillometry measurements and ventricular volume in patients with aneurysmal subarachnoid hemorrhage. *J Neurosci Nurs.* 2022; 54: 166–70.

355. K Giamarino, SS Reynolds. Pupillometry in neurocritical care. *Nursing.* 2022; 52: 41–4.

356. A Kamal, KM Ahmed, AM Venkatachalam, M Osman, SG Aoun, V Aiyagari, et al. Pilot study of neurologic pupil index as a predictor of external ventricular drain clamp trial failure after subarachnoid hemorrhage. *World Neurosurg.* 2022; 164: 2–7.

357. JG Kim, H Shin, TH Lim, W Kim, Y Cho, BH Jang, et al. Efficacy of quantitative pupillary light reflex for predicting neurological outcomes in patients treated with targeted temperature management after cardiac arrest: A systematic review and meta-analysis. *Medicina Kaunas.* 2022; 58: 804.

358. CH Wang, CY Wu, CC Liu, TC Hsu, MA Liu, MC Wu, et al. Neuroprognostic accuracy of quantitative versus standard pupillary light reflex for adult postcardiac arrest patients: A systematic review and meta-analysis. *Crit Care Med.* 2021; 49: 1790–9.

359. B Thakur, H Nadim, F Atem, SE Stutzman, DM Olson. Dilation velocity is associated with Glasgow Coma Scale scores in patients with brain injury. *Brain Inj.* 2021; 35: 114–18.

360. C Sandroni, G Citerio, FS Taccone. Automated pupillometry in intensive care. *Intens Care Med.* 2022; 48: 1467–70.

361. P Lenga, D Kuhlwein, S Schonenberger, JO Neumann, AW Unterberg, C Beynon. The use of quantitative pupillometry in brain death determination: Preliminary findings. *Neurol Sci.* 2023. Accession Number: 38082049. Published online.

362. L Kelvin. *Popular Lectures and Addresses*, Vol. 1. London: Macmillan; 1889.

Index